HEALTH AND STRENGTH

MAGAZINE

NOVEMBER 1900

FACSIMILE REPRODUCTION

HEALTH AND STRENGTH

MAGAZINE

NOVEMBER 1900

FACSIMILE REPRODUCTION

Alan Stuart Radley

RADLEY

BOOKS

2018

for

Mum And Dad

and dedicated to:

David Gentle, Kim Veltman, Francisco, Restie and
Rowena, Ruth and Chris, and Philip, Ellen, Nigel,
Arlene, Joshua, Emma, Ben and Caroline Radley.

HEALTH & STRENGTH

HOW "STRONG ARM" BECAME CHIEF OF THE IROQUOIS.

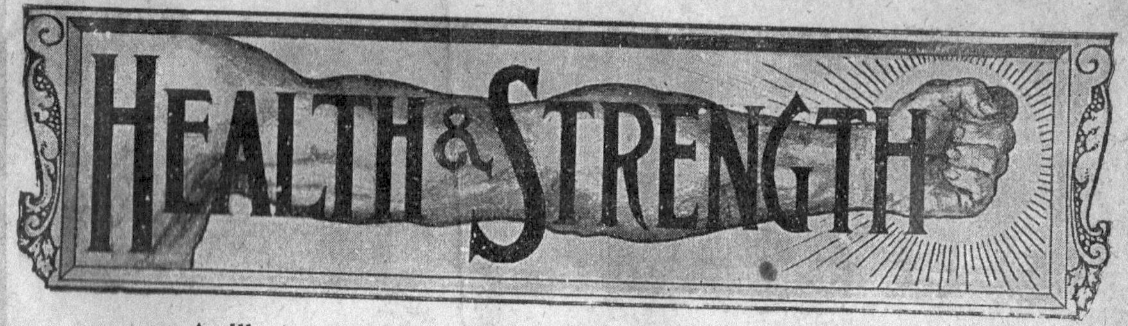

An Illustrated Monthly Magazine devoted to subjects appertaining to
HEALTH, STRENGTH, VITALITY, MUSCULAR DEVELOPMENT, FOOD, CLOTHING, AND THE GENERAL CARE OF THE BODY
Copyright Registered at Stationers' Hall.

No. 8. Vol. II.   **Price 3/- per Year, Postfree.**   NOVEMBER, 1900.

IMPORTANT NOTICE.

Registered Cable and Telegraphic Address: "*Herculean, London.*"

Editorial communications should be addressed The Editor, HEALTH & STRENGTH MONTHLY, 73, Farringdon Street, London, E.C.

Business letters should be addressed The Manager.

Cheques and P.O. Orders should be crossed "Economic Bank," and made payable to THE HEALTH AND STRENGTH Co.

Remittances from abroad must be by Money Order.

Subscription. 3/- per annum. Foreign, 4/-

Publishing Day.—Fifteenth of month.

Advertising.—Matter for advertisements must be received not later than 1st of month.

ADVERTISEMENT RATES:
Small Advertisements

1d. per word. Four insertions at price of three.

Display Advertisements:

(Alongside reading matter).	£	s.	d.
2nd or 4th p. of Cover, per insertion	5	0	0
Half ,, ,, ,,	3	0	0
Quarter ,, ,, ,,	2	0	0
Eighth ,, ,, ,,	1	5	0
3rd p. of Cover, per insertion	4	0	0
Half ,, ,, ,,	2	10	0
Quarter ,, ,,	1	10	0
Eighth ,, ,,	1	0	0
Other pages, per insertion	3	0	0
Half ,, ,, ,,	1	15	0
Quarter ,, ,,	1	0	0
Eighth ,, ,,	0	15	0
Per inch (among reading matter on pages 2, 3, 4, 5 or 7)	0	7	6

Discount for series of insertions: 5 % on 3, 10 % on 6, and 15 % on 12 insertions respectively.

Advts. of Tobaccos, Cigarettes, Cigars, Alcoholic Liquors and "Cure-All" Medicines not accepted.

Scathing Condemnation of Modern Medical Butchers.

BY J. H. GREER, M.D.

What a field for butchery and for the attainment of fame and money woman has become to the mercenary practitioner of so-called 'modern gynecology' (female diseases). It would be interesting, were it not revolting, to trace the history of the treatment of diseases of women by the majority of the medical profession during the past twenty years.

"Some of the fads profitably encouraged by the medical profession are not only absurd, but are almost criminal in their methods.

"Little do the fathers and husbands and brothers know of the indignities their daughters or wives or sisters are often forced to endure in the way of uncalled-for exposures and mutilations to satisfy the notions and mercenary appetites of modern gynecologists.

"My large experience in all diseases of women has brought to my knowledge thousands of cases where women and virgins have been needlessly subjected to revolting exposures and painful operations, only to be mutilated for life and left in a far worse condition than when they applied for relief.

"Who can enumerate the cases in which the abdomen has been opened for supposed ovarian diseases when not a trace of a pathological (diseased) condition was discoverable? Who will write the history of the cases in which perfectly healthy ovaries have been removed without one shadow of improvement in the general condition of the patient? A human being mutilated, deprived of her distinctive characteristics, and rendered miserable! A human life poised between earth and heaven to gratify ignorance or conceit! A human life sacrificed to ambition upon the operating table!

"When it is of almost daily occurrence for me to be consulted by those who were on the verge of submitting to wholly needless and brutal mutilations, and for me to start them on the road to recovery by the employment of rational means, I feel justified in saying, in the name of womanhood, in the name of common honesty, in the name of humanity, defend yourselves, your wives, your daughters, your sisters and your friends from the hands of the professional mutilators of women."

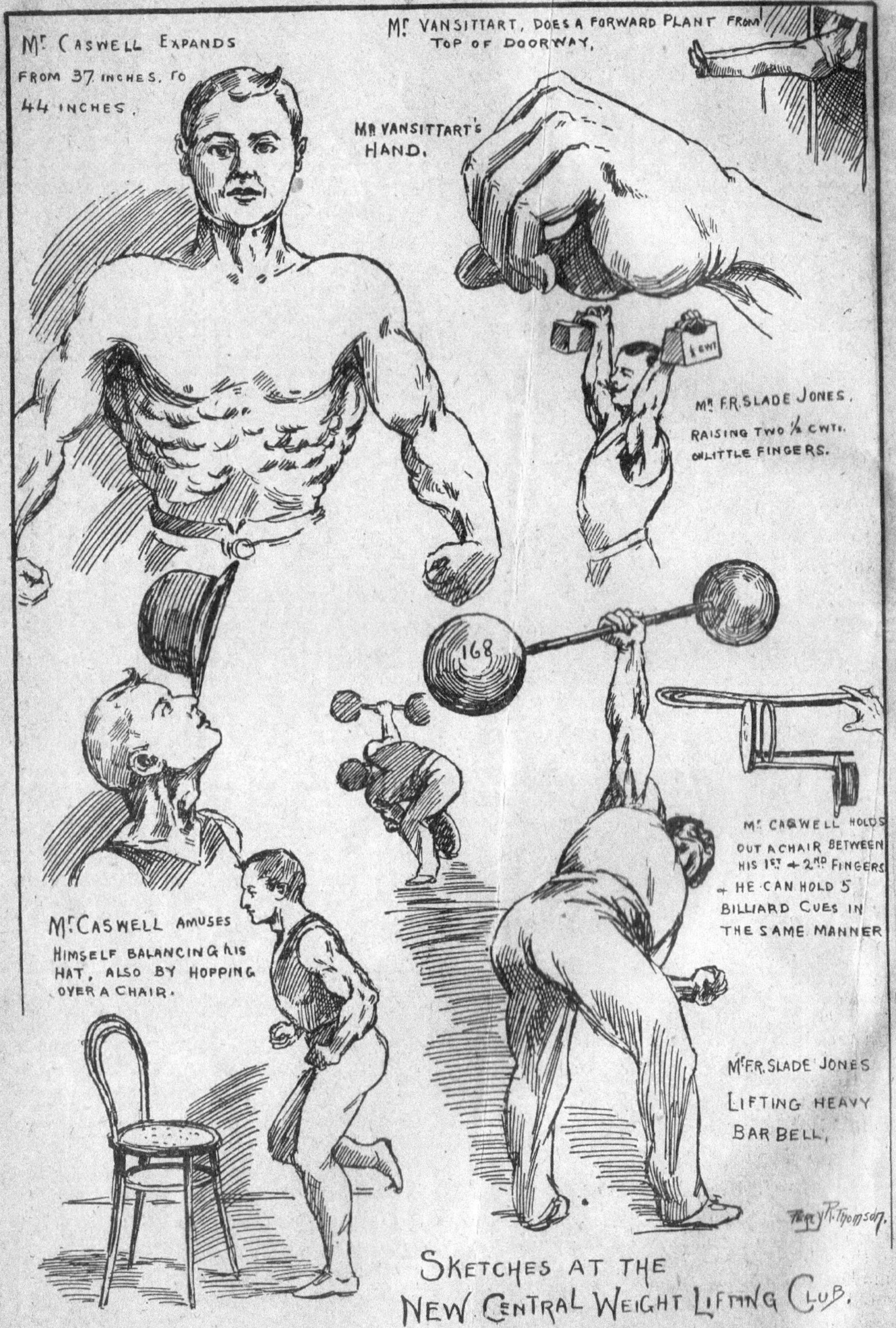

M? CASWELL EXPANDS FROM 37 INCHES. TO 44 INCHES.
M? VANSITTART, DOES A FORWARD PLANT FROM TOP OF DOORWAY.
MR VANSITTART'S HAND.
M? F.R. SLADE JONES. RAISING TWO ½ CWT. ON LITTLE FINGERS.
168
M? CASWELL HOLDS OUT A CHAIR BETWEEN HIS 1ST & 2ND FINGERS & HE CAN HOLD 5 BILLIARD CUES IN THE SAME MANNER
M? CASWELL AMUSES HIMSELF BALANCING HIS HAT, ALSO BY HOPPING OVER A CHAIR.
M? F.R. SLADE JONES LIFTING HEAVY BAR BELL.
SKETCHES AT THE NEW CENTRAL WEIGHT LIFTING CLUB.

Holidays for Business Men.

A gentleman, high in the councils of a great corporation, told me yesterday that for fifteen years he had not been away from his office, that for fifteen years he had been trying unavailingly to find time to visit Del Monte—a four hours' trip from San Francisco. I am thinking seriously of starting a petition in an endeavour to get the governor to pardon him out. I don't know what his crime was, but fifteen years in confinement at hard labour entitles him to parole long enough to become acquainted with the rising and setting sun.

This is one of our later day manias that must be reckoned with if our business establishments are not to be turned into hospitals and insane asylums. Factories, offices, buildings, stores—they are prisons of humanity, confined by circumstance. This confinement is sometimes the result of seeming necessity, but very often it is the result of inertia, or of a most narrow and ignorant view as to what constitutes success, or misapprehension of the purpose of ambition. In many cases inertia is at fault—"too much trouble to take a vacation." It is like stirring up a bear in midwinter—"what's the use of getting up." As for the man who believes himself indispensable to any office, any profession, any business, I need but say that while all manner of indefensible praise has been inscribed on helpless monuments, no one has yet had the hardihood to write, "Here lies Mr. Double Blank, he was indispensable to the earth." Therefore, get away. Go somewhere. Go where the only ceiling is a blue sky, where the walls are tree-decked mountains, counters running streams, desks great boulders, and the pavements but trails. At home the telephone and telegraph are your masters; when you are away refer them to the red-headed woodpecker in the highest pine tree. Go away to some place where you can dispense with starch, both in your clothing and your manners, without occasioning criticism. If you have not been in prison so long as to be afraid of a moonlit sky and the wide expanse of the universe to which you were born heir, have you not eyes? Sleep out of doors. If you are not too dulled by electric lights to lose the glory of a camp fire, build one and remember that Prometheus did not recommend an oil stove. Put on the clothes that will make you feel most at home when you lean up against a tree, and try drinking out of a spring instead of a bottle. Go away to the mountains or to the shore. If Adam had been a housed-up man like you, poring over routine details, of which many are not instructive at all, even though interesting; if he had spent his life facing a lot of pigeon-holes, and his example had been followed by descendants obedient to precedent, it's a pretty specimen of a man you would be to-day. You couldn't go anywhere—you might be shipped by express. If three months of every year's time can be spent in the open air, very good; you do a year's work in the other nine; if but one month or one week, take that. You cannot go wrong if you go for but a day. But come out of your sarcophagus and take a vacation. You are entitled to it, and what is of more importance, the people who must associate with you are entitled to it. Take a vacation for their sake if not your own.—*Sunset.*

Rhymes of Man, Mule and Goat.

By S. E. KISER.

LORDLY MAN AND LOWLY MULE.

Man is the greatest work of God,
  The oxen are his slaves;
He lures the lightning from the cloud,
  And harnesses the waves.

To him alone a soul is given,
  And he receives at birth
The glorious hope of joy in heaven
  When he is done with earth.

Man is sublime, the homely mule
  Is made of poorer stuff,
But mules quit drinking, as a rule,
  When they have had enough.

MAN THE GODLIKE, GOAT THE MEAN.

The goat is not regarded as
  A noble beast, and it
Has never won distinction for
  An undue share of wit.

Compare the homely goat with man:
  How Godlike does he stand;
How pitiful the beast becomes
  And how absurdly planned!

Yet, while we look upon the goat
  As neither fair nor wise,
It doesn't live by taking pills
  Instead of exercise.

The Strongest Man in the World.

Refused Life Insurance when 19.
Took up Physical Culture, and now Breaks Horse-shoes
and Forged Steel Chains and Bars.

THE MOST MARVELLOUS DEVELOPMENT EVER SEEN.
(Illustrated by Photos taken exclusively for "Health and Strength.")

The above startling statements are a true titular introduction to an article about one who, had he been the original of "The Village Blacksmith," would have caused the author to substitute "stronger than" for "strong as" the "iron bands" to which he likened the muscles of his hero knight of the anvil.

his premiums. Yet such was the experience of Mr Vansittart when 19 years of age.

Probably, had Mr. Vansittart been accepted by the insurance company—passing even by the skin of his teeth, so to speak,—he might never have thought of taking up Physical Culture, so true is it that the majority of us

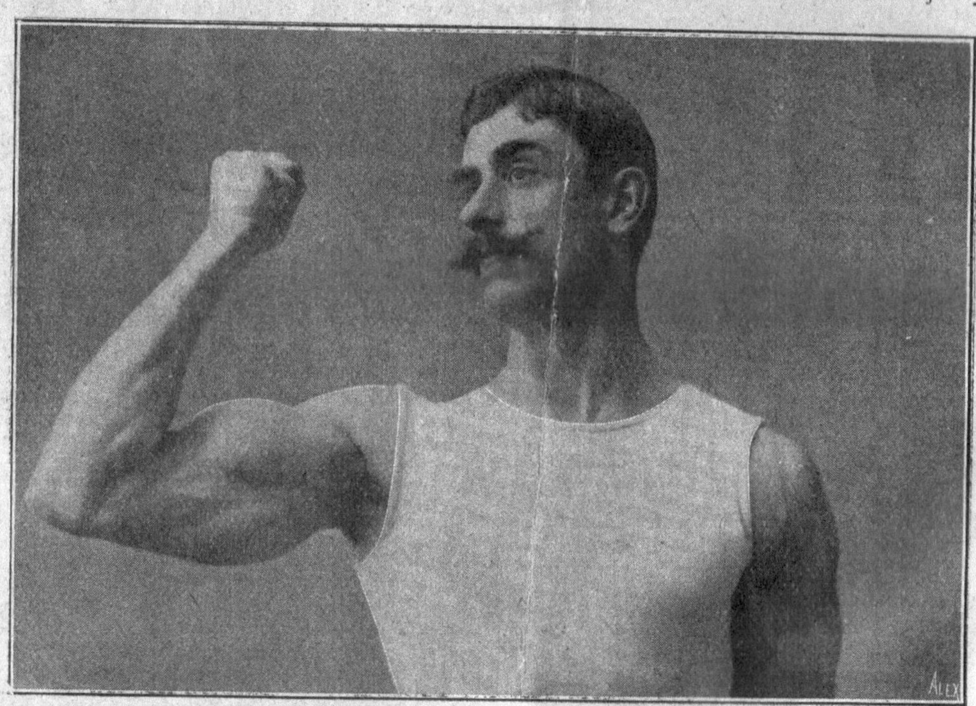

MR. VANSITTART'S WONDERFUL RIGHT ARM.

Mr. Charles (the writer was so overawed by the size of his muscles as to quite forget to ask for his other extra names) Vansittart furnishes a striking example of what may be accomplished by those who—however weak and unhealthy they may be—will only persevere with Physical Culture. A man has to be a pretty likely candidate for an early funeral to be refused by an insurance company. He must have one leg in the grave, and that properly in, to fail to pass the doctor in a class of business in which the paid officials from the manager downwards have a monetary interest in putting him on their books and receiving

have to be frightened into doing a thing which, to be done well, requires more than a little sticking to. Therefore, let us take unto ourselves the moral that if we are not as weak as others, we ought nevertheless to make ourselves as strong and healthy as possible.

We may conclude (he did not say so) that Mr. Vansittart was frightened into trying to repair his health and strength—anyway he did try, and with so great a measure of success that in the time of the memorable Klondyke boom he felt strong and healthy enough to brave the hardships of that notoriously rough quarter of the world. His health and strength stood the severe test, and, indeed, enabled him to make money.

Then occurred an unfortunate mine speculation in which he lost all the money he had made, together with other money which represented his private income for two-thirds of the ensuing year.

Here was an awkward fix, and the prospect looked as black as only a Klondyke winter, with the most necessary articles of food selling at fabulous prices, can look. Probably actuated by an unconscious desire for the sympathy of human companionship, he unconsciously strolled into a typical Klondyke resort—half music hall and half public house orpheum. Here the "star" attraction was a "Strong Man," whose feats our hero had a somewhat hazy idea he would equal. He must have said as much to some of the by-

At one place a noted local blacksmith spent a whole day in forging and re-forging a special horse-shoe. He challenged Mr. Vansittart to break it, and said he would give him $50 if he broke it. This was the toughest job of Mr. Vansittart's whole professional career. For half-an-hour he toiled over it—but he did it, and secured the reward, the blacksmith generously adding a full measure of praise for a feat which he believed to be absolutely impossible.

A man challenged the genuineness of Mr. Vansittart's feats at Seattle, and foolishly did more by insulting him. Mr. Vansittart not inexcusably lost his temper (he did not strike me as having one at all, so quiet and modest is he), and gripping his insulter by his neck and the seat of his unmentionables threw him into the orchestra. The man had nothing more to say.

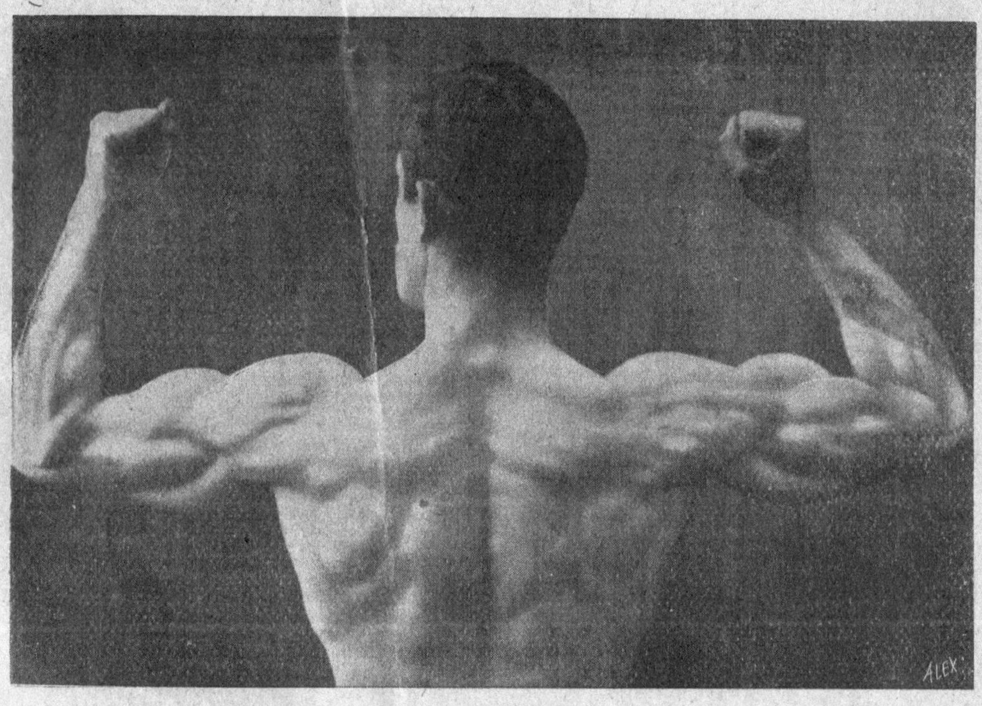

HE IS A LIVING MUSCULAR CHART.

standers, for arrangements were made for him to prove himself as good as he thought he was.

First he essayed the "Strong Man's" feat of holding hands gripped together with two men pulling ropes round each upper arm. This proved easy, and more and more men were added until 20 was the number of men he found he could withstand.

Mr. Vansittart did the Strong Man business in Seattle, Portland, Spokane, Rossland, etc., his feats growing even more marvellous as his strength grew.

With harness he lifted the heaviest horse that could be produced, he raised a 250-lb. bar-bell, tore three packs of cards at once, broke horse-shoes, bolts and "tenpenny" nails.

The Chief Inspector of Police at Victoria, British Columbia, possesses a unique memento of Mr. Vansittart's strength. He prided himself on a special make of handcuffs, and challenged Mr. Vansittart to break through them. Mr. Vansittart gives the official credit for some justification for his pride, but he broke them after a stiff struggle. I might add that Mr. Vansittart states that the ordinary handcuffs are no bar to his liberty, and at the London Alhambra broke a pair one night when Houdini was exhibiting.

By-the-bye, Mr. Vansittart emphatically discredits the "feats" of one or two "Strong Men" who claim to break coins. The coins that are broken are specially prepared, and he suggested that placing a coin in a vice and attempting to bend it with sharp blows with a hammer will convince the average man that it is not possible to bend a normal coin with the fingers.

On the other hand, Mr. Vansittart occasionally comes across a man who discredits everything.

Mr. Vansittart asked at the bar for a couple of packs and did the two together before the astonished eyes of the rash challenger, who no doubt now has a paraphrase of his own of the phrase that one sometimes entertains angels (or strong men) unaware. The amusing part about this particular incident was that the man

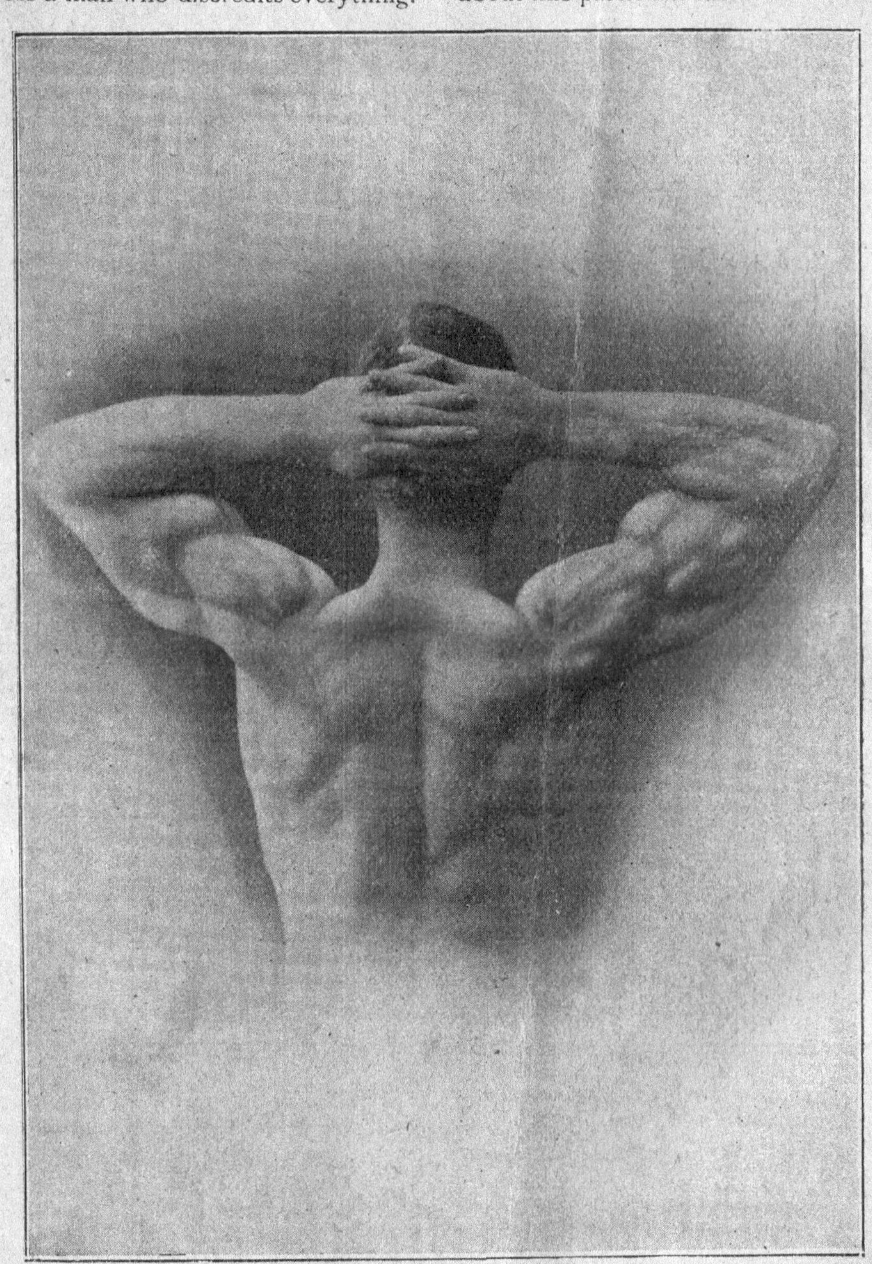

NOTE THE FINE DELTOIDS AND TRICEPS.

At a place of entertainment in London the other day a man loudly discredited the feat of tearing a single pack of cards. Mr. Vansittart took up the defence of the strong man who had just done the feat by saying it was possible. The man replied that he would believe it when he saw Mr. Vansittart do it, and offered to bet him £5 that he could not do a single pack.

bet more money than he had upon him—thirty shillings being his all, and which Mr. Vansittart refused to accept from a sad if a wiser man.

Mr. Vansittart has lifted a 259-lb. bar-bell, and while holding it aloft allowed two men to get atop. the whole of which weight he thus supported. He is 6-ft. 1-in., and not what I should term broad in proportion, but he does a "front plant" (see sketches on another page of scenes at Central Weight-Lifting Club.) I also saw him do an upward plant off his shoulders on the floor whilst grasping a 250-lb. bar-bell. He has "pulled up" on the rings with 90-lb. weight attached to himself.

A special feat of one strong man in America was to support a 1-in. diameter and 18 x 16-ft. iron bar on his head, with hands to steady, and whilst eight people simultaneously put the whole of their weight at each end, to bend the rod. This Mr. Vansittart beat by bending the same diameter rod, but only 6-ft. long, and without the weight leverage of a single person, by pulling on the rod with both hands and using his head as the fulcrum.

flexing the biceps and triceps muscle. Readers may detect a difference in the muscles of the two upper arm muscles. This was caused by the breaking of one of the right arm muscles during the execution of this feat. Fortunately the muscle joined and healed in a way which did not affect its strength.

Mr. Vansittart has a truly marvellous chest expansion, viz., 9 inches—that is, difference between chest empty and fully inflated. He can also expand his neck $1\frac{1}{2}$ inches and let four people pull a noose on it.

He is 32 years of age, his weight $12\frac{1}{2}$ stone, upper arm $17\frac{3}{4}$, forearm 14, wrist $7\frac{1}{4}$.

I might write a lot more about Mr. Vansittart —even about things I have seen him do —but

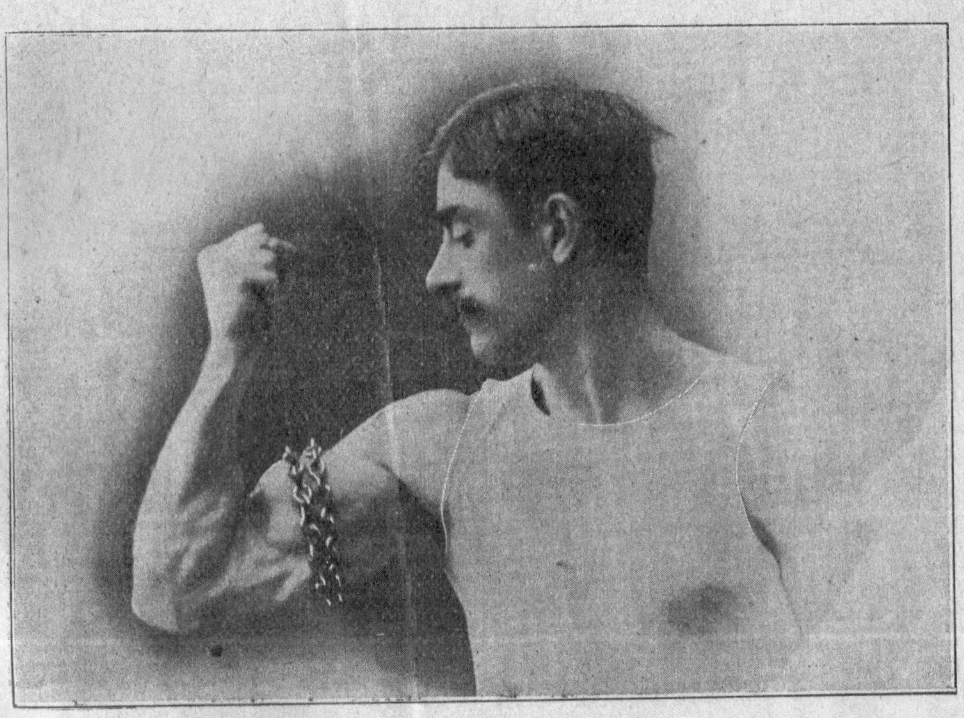

HE BREAKS CHAINS LIKE STRING.

He has never had his special feats beaten. He has amused himself at country house parties by picking up the balls whilst tennis is in progress and bursting them in his hands, (readers might try this for themselves—it won't cost much to buy the new balls that will be needed). The players would be puzzled to account for the way in which the balls all seemed to go wrong. They would search the tennis racquets for nails or other things likely to cause the trouble, but would remain puzzled until Mr. Vansittart chose to enlighten them.

Another good feat of Mr. Vansittart's is to bend a $\frac{3}{8}$-in. iron ring round upper arm by

I will publish them at some future time. I am much indebted—and I am sure my readers will join me in thanks to him—to Mr. Vansittart for his kindness in having these latest photos taken purposely for this article. Another and closer view of Mr. Vansittart will appear in the next (Xmas) number. I might add that the photos, as also a huge forged steel nail, bent in my presence, is on view at the office of this magazine, and readers are invited to call and inspect them, as also photos of other strong men—professional and amateur.

The photos illustrating this article are by Messrs. W. & J. Stuart, 47 & 49, Brompton Road, S.W.

Experiences of Physical Culture.

The Editor would like to hear from those who, like himself, have been brought from extreme weakness to health and strength through Physical Culture. It encourages others in their endeavours to improve their physical condition. Whenever possible please send photographs.

Before Training could only lift 36-lbs., but can now lift 123 lbs.

HIGH STREET, SLOUGH.

DEAR SIR,—Although I cannot claim that Physical Culture has actually cured me of any disease, I think that my experiences may prove of some help to others.

Like a large number of others my weakness was the chief thing that made me begin. Although I was then $17\frac{1}{2}$ years of age I could only lift 36-lbs. with one hand and 56-lbs. with two (over my head of course). I bought one of Sandow's books and commenced the exercises. These, with certain alterations, I kept up for a year. Since that period I have only used india-rubber. My health has improved greatly, and my measurements, as well as my actual strength, have greatly increased. Several other fellows round here have started and are getting on famously. My measurements and lifting powers are:—

MEASUREMENTS.

	Before Training.		Present.
Age	$17\frac{1}{2}$	...	$19\frac{1}{2}$
Chest normal ...	33	...	40
,, expanded ...	36	...	42
Biceps (flexed) ...	$11\frac{1}{4}$	...	15
Forearm	10	...	12
Thigh	18	...	$21\frac{1}{2}$
Calf	13	...	14

LIFTING.

	Before Training.		Present.
Right hand ...	36-lbs.	...	123-lbs,
Left hand ...	33-lbs.	...	100-lbs.
Both hands ...	56-lbs.	...	150-lbs.

Photograph enclosed.—Sincerely yours,

T. HERBERT.

Never felt better in my Life.

I herewith testify that since I have used your Exerciser I never felt better in my life, Before I started I was going very thin, couldn't sleep at nights, and no strength at all; in fact I was in a very weak state and had to consult a doctor, but I am very pleased to say I need no doctor now, thanks to your grand Health Exerciser. All my friends who saw me when I started can hardly believe their own eyes when they see the improvement in me. I gave my heart and soul to it, and stuck to it VERY HARD, and mastered all the EXERCISES. I know several fellows who use your Exerciser, but they use it only a few times—they remark it is too much like hard work. I tell them what I think of anyone making such a child's remark. When I show photo they won't believe it is me. I tell them it was a PLEASURE to me to use the Exerciser, and that they would develop the same way if they followed your instructions. G. B. BUSTIN, BRISTOL (*whose photo appeared in the August issue*).

IVY COTTAGE, MERTHYR, S. WALES,

... I am very pleased with MONTHLY, and will willingly pay 2d. for future numbers as I think they are well worth it for the good advice they give. I wish you every success. You deserve to be more widely known for the good you are doing.

GEO. SISSONS,

Hoping that it will be a greater success than ever.

A. F. FRAZER, PERTH.

For Young Men from a Young Man.

I have read with keen interest the various experiences given in our valuable little Monthly. All experience, when it is that of honest folk, is instructive, and when the aim is to make others sharers in what we ourselves have found to be a blessing, then our motive in communicating our experience is much to be commended.

Very early in life I began to have notions about, and to admire, beauty and symmetry of the human form. Although not of robust health myself, I used to frequent the gymnasium, if not to do much exercise on the apparatus myself, to see others and admire and envy their beautifully developed bodies, and in a quiet way I determined to have a stronger body, and set myself to study how this could be acquired. "The Boy's book of Health and Strength," by Dr. Gordon Stables, of "B.O.P." fame, gave me some of my first lessons in health and proper care of the body. This is a book that every boy should have in his library—especially sons of Scotia, as it is decidedly a Scotch book, and the reading of it cannot but interest those who, like myself, are Scotch and brought up on "parritch, halesome food o' Scotia's sons." Sandow's dumb-bell system and book next came under notice, and I worked away with great expectations, but the development promised failed to appear. What is wrong with the system is the use of too heavy bells and continued tension. I had reached dumb-bells of 7-lbs. when I ceased. A display by Professor B. A. Macfadden attracted me at this time, and his "Physical Training" was purchased and read with interest. What young man, after reading the essay in the book: "For the Young Man," but is enthused with the earnest appeal and sincerity of the writer. Is there a reader of "H. & S." who does not yet possess this book? Get it at once, and an Exerciser along with it. I was always a bit of a faddist, but after reading "Physical Training" I developed quite into a Mac-fad-denist. I was soon the happy possessor of a Style A Exerciser, and from time to time have added to my stock every appliance which bears his name. I believe in variety when exercising. "Fifteen minutes with dumb-bells followed by a cold bath" is far too monotonous, and, if we wish a well-developed and symmetrical body, all sorts of exercise should be engaged in, and interest kept up by variety. The term Physical Culture is generally only applied to exercise of the muscular system, but in its broadest sense it means much more, viz., whatever tends to cultivate, strengthen, or beautify man's body, "the temple of the soul," and, if this is the object, remember the essentials—"be persistent in your exercise and strong in your determination to reach the goal." Pure air, pure food and drink, pure morals; temperate in all things, and there is no doubt but that you will realize your ideal.

Yours for health and strength,

WILLIAM M. SCOTT.

Townhill, Dumfermline.

I should like to say, here, that I think yours an excellent paper, and I am doing my best to make it known personally. I have derived much benefit from physical culture. I firmly believe dumb-bells and cold baths have cured me of biliousness, and also cleared my complexion of blotches, blackheads, etc. With best wishes, H. L. A., MEDHURST.

Am very pleased with your Friction Towel; it is splendid after the cold tub.

C. H. WILKINSON, EASTBOURNE.

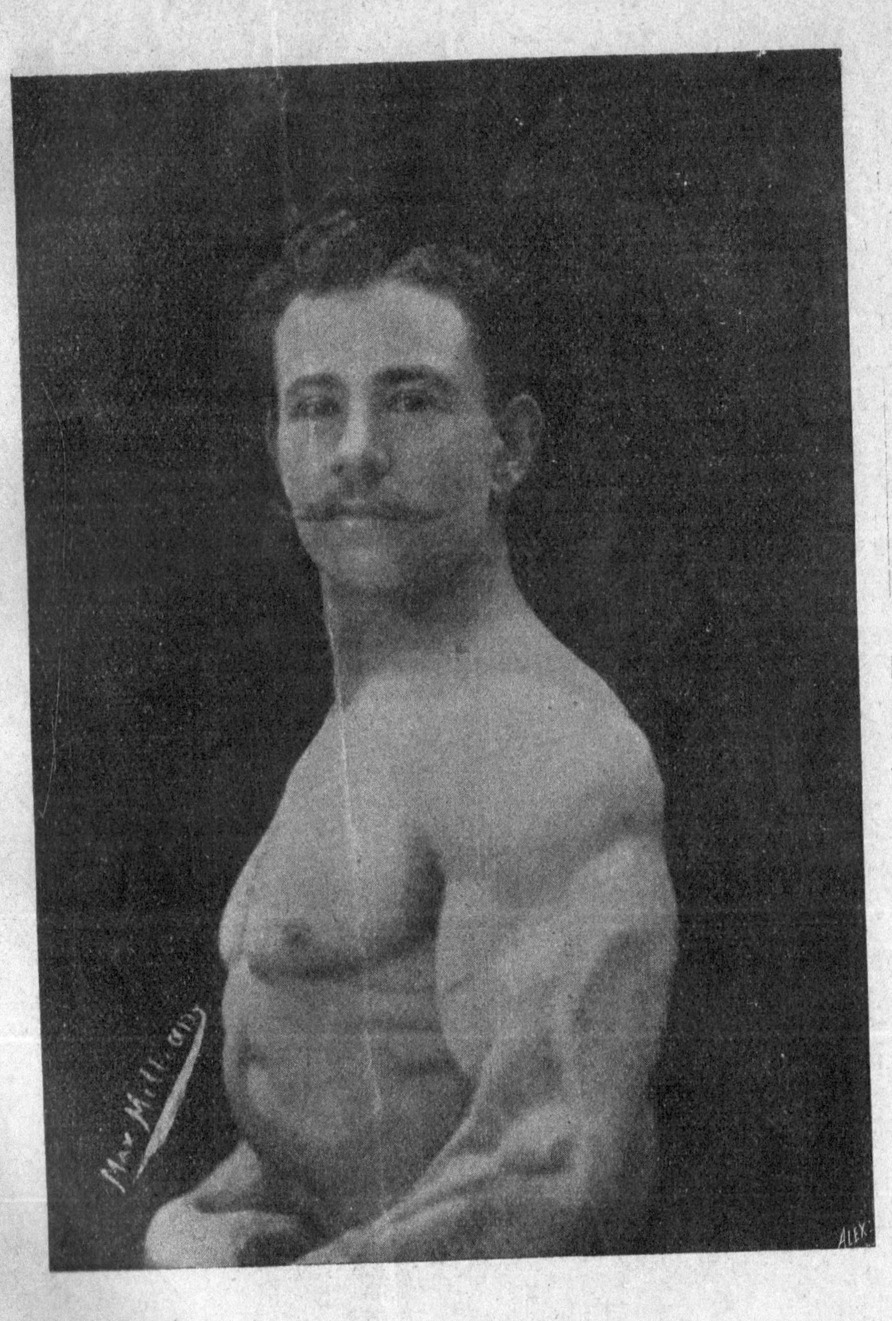

MAX MILIAN.

A FINE LEFT ARM.

(Photo by F. Porcher & Co.)

Tricks and Tests of Muscle.

By "Wrestler."

["Tricks and Tests of Muscle" will now be a regular feature of Health & Strength. Every reader who becomes acquainted with, and practices, them will be a welcome acquisition wherever two or three healthy and strong young men are gathered together. Unlike many forms of recreation, the "tricks and tests of muscle" will benefit the participants in health and strength. Readers will greatly oblige by drawing the attention of their friends to this interesting feature of Health & Strength. "Tricks and Tests of Muscle" commenced in May issue. If you know any "Tricks and Tests of Muscle" kindly send them along to "The Wrestler."

— The Editor.]

Finger Flexibility Test.

The pianist or violinist is about the most likely person to succeed with this usually impossible test. Bend the second finger of both hands, as shown in sketch, and place knuckles

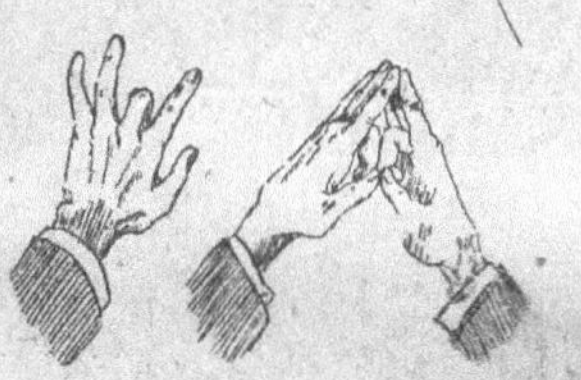

one against the other, and ends of fingers and thumbs, as shown in second sketch. The test is to see if you can keep the second joints of the two bent second fingers close together whilst holding ends of other fingers and thumbs together.

Body Muscles Test.

This is a very severe test of the body muscles, including those of the neck, back, chest, abdomen, and legs and feet. Some of my readers will no doubt have seen this feat performed at mesmeric entertainments, where, however, the ability to do it was ascribed to mesmeric influence. The best way to practice

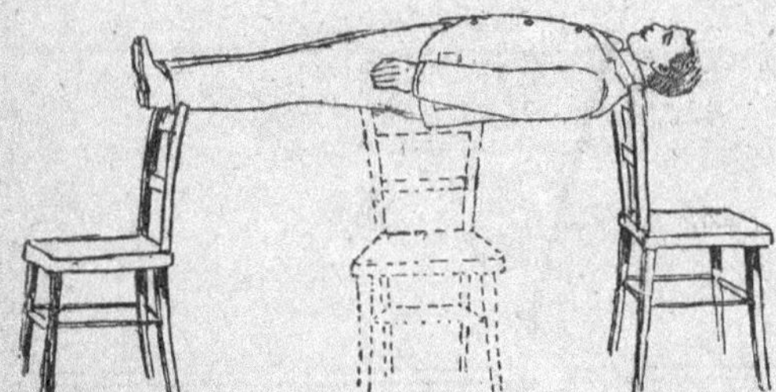

this at first is to use a table instead of chairs, for the neck and ankles using rests made of suitable blocks of wood. If the body can then be held above the table the performer may then to essay feat proper, getting a friend

to afford a start by placing a chair as shown by dotted lines, and then at your word of command withdrawing same. Until the performer has perfect control over muscles that are strong enough to do the feat without any trouble, he had better pave the way for a rapid descent with cushions or similar fall-breakers.

Grip and Arm Muscle Test.

See who can hold out at arm's length the heaviest chair in the way illustrated. Many

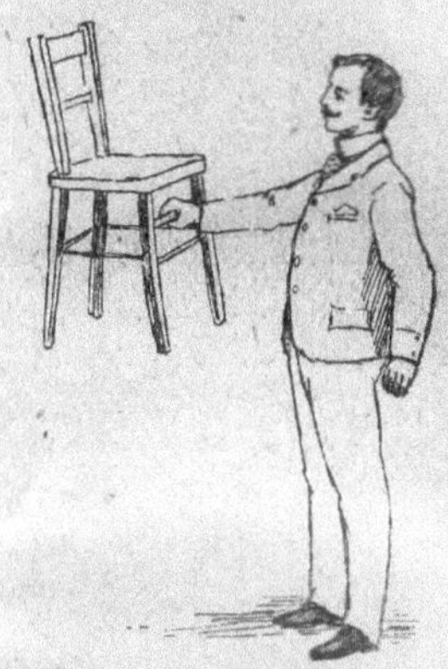

men who can lift big weights in a way which makes no great call for strength of grip, fail miserably where a strong grip is required. The arm muscles are always stronger than those of the wrist, hand and and fingers, and the finest thing I know of for developing great strength in these weaker muscles are the Grip Machines sold by the Health and Strength Co., at 2/3 (wood handles) and 4/3 (cork handles). They are certainly wonderful value to anyone who desires to make the weaker muscles stronger,

(To be continued in our next issue.)

Special.

[Those who would like to be fully prepared with "100 Tricks and Tests of Muscle" should send order at once for the new book under that title by "Wrestler," and which will be published in a few days by the Health and Strength Co. at 1/- net. The book will have over 100 illustrations, and "The Wrestler" desires me to inform readers that all who send 1/- Postal Orders before Dec. 1st. will receive book (post free) specially bound, and containing photos of various strong men. Don't wait until the last day of the month before sending, or something may crop up to prevent your order reaching "The Wrestler" in time. There will be only a limited number of this specially bound edition, and orders will be booked and despatched exactly as received. —The Ed.]

Weights and Measures.

By F. Williamson.

A great deal of harm has been done, and is being done, by professional "strong men" and others who profess to lift enormous weights, which in many cases are not one-half the weight they are supposed to be. At the present time so much interest is taken in Physical Culture, and so many boys and young men are taking it up, that unless they know what standards and records to aim at they are likely to do themselves more harm than good by their efforts.

A young man after seeing one of the numerous strong men perform often becomes filled with enthusiasm to emulate his feats, and forthwith begins to practice vigorously. At the end of twelve months he finds, perhaps, that he can elevate a 56-lb. weight in each hand simultaneously, if so he is getting along very nicely, for not one in a thousand can do this feat, simple as it sounds. But as a rule the novice does not know this, and having seen the performer raise 350-lbs. or so in one hand, he begins to think he is not cut out for the strong man business, and gives up in despair, Nil desperandum should be his motto.

The best criterion of what can be accomplished in lifting heavy weights is shown by the feats performed by the Amateur Champion, Launceston Elliott, who last year in the competition for the championship lifted 205-lbs. with the left hand, and 215-lbs. with the right. With two hands he lifted 245½-lbs., using two separate dumb-bells, whilst with a bar-bell he lifted 265-lbs. These are amazing feats, and it is not too much to say that not one of the professional "strong men" at present before the public could accomplish them. When you see a performer lifting anything stated to be beyond 250-lbs., have the weight weighed before believing it to be genuine.

If a man can lift one hundred-weight with one hand, or a bar-bell weighing 150-lbs. with two hands, he may consider himself very fair; he will be able to hold his own in respectable company.

In regard to measurements almost as much misconception prevails. One man says he can expand his chest to 56 inches, whereupon another goes one better and says he can expand to 60, and so on. Thus the old fable of the frog and bull is repeated, and perhaps in time will end in the same manner by one of them bursting. If a man reaches 40 inches round the chest he is big; if he can stretch the tape to 45 he is exceptional, so that you can see what the above figures are worth.

Then again the tape measure is no gauge of a man's strength. Take two men of the same age, one weighing 13-st. and the other 10-st., it does not follow that the bigger and heavier is the stronger. In many cases the smaller, and to all appearances the weaker, man is far stronger than the big man. These things show that mere size is nothing without a strong will and plenty of nerve force to back it up.

Again, in two men who have almost exactly the same measurements, there is often a great difference in weight. In a recent number of Health and Strength there appeared an interview with Mr. Slade-Jones which gave measurements. A friend of the writer's has almost the same measurements as Mr. Jones, yet he scales a stone-and-a-half more. This is accounted for by the fact that one has bigger and heavier bones, which could be shown by taking the measurements of the joints, viz., the wrist, elbow, knee and ankle.

Apollo, who is one of the honestest men on the stage, gives it as his opinion that a man cannot expand his chest more than two or three inches above the normal. Of course, between the contracted chest and the fully expanded chest there are many who can show a difference of from six to eight inches, but to measure the chest at its normal size, that is, as a man carries it without strain, and then when expanded to its utmost, the difference is very slight. Apollo candidly states that 250-lbs. is as much as any man can lift, and any statement beyond that he is very sceptical about.

If the reader of Health and Strength takes all the foregoing points into consideration, he will be more satisfied with the result of his work. He should remember that Physical Culture is not a sport like football, which can only be followed for a few years, nor is it a three months' course at a gymnasium, but something to be taken daily as inevitably as one's food. Bearing this in mind, the pupil will go slowly but far.

***

Mr. Grandhi, a Hindoo teacher, when asked if vegetarianism did not impair the strength, silenced his interested questioners by saying that when the meat-eating Englishman went to India, the rice-eating coolie had to carry him! And when both were wounded in battle, he of the purer diet recovered far more quickly from his injury.

Sometime ago there was a walking test of endurance near Berlin between eight vegetarians and fourteen meat-eaters. All the vegetarians, save two, reached the goal first, fresh and in fine condition—while one meat-eater only arrived, one hour later, quite exhausted—his confrères having one by one fallen out on the way.

Wrestling.

BY PERCY LONGHURST,

Light Weight Amateur Champion (C. & W. Style) 1900.
Winner Light Weight Competition, German Gynasium Society Competitions, 1899.
Late Leader of Wrestling, Orion Gymnastic Club.

PART II.

THE FLYING MAZE.

This is properly a Cornish throw, and is very useful and effective.

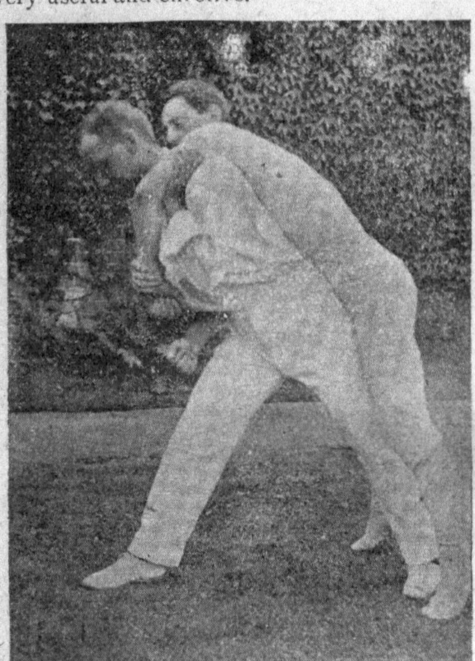

THE FLYING MAZE.

Seize the left wrist in your right hand, turn your back to the man, stooping slightly, gripping his upper left arm in your left hand thus bringing his arm over your left shoulder ; you may now throw him clean over your back, with or without the assistance of the legs ; but great quickness is necessary to stop, seiz tightly round the body with the free arm and throw the man forward on his face by clutching his legs.

I may say here, by the way, that catch-hold wrestlers, as a rule, neglect to use their feet and legs far too much, thereby placing themselves at a disadvantage, and they place far too much reliance on ground wrestling, which is largely a matter of weight and strength.

THROW FROM ONE LEG.

Dash in and obtain hold of one thigh, low down, try and lift from the floor, and click the other leg from the inside very low down with your opposite foot, throwing the man a clean fall backwards. The hold cannot always be obtained straight away, but the opportunity frequently presents itself while wrestling. If your opponent get the hold on you and insert the click you are lost ; if you cannot release your leg turn and fall on your face before he get in the click.

WRIST AND THIGH THROW.

Seize left wrist in right hand, step in with left foot and head low, catching the left thigh in your left arm and drawing his captured hand backwards, lift clear of the ground and swing his legs to the left ; he is now lying across your neck and shoulders.

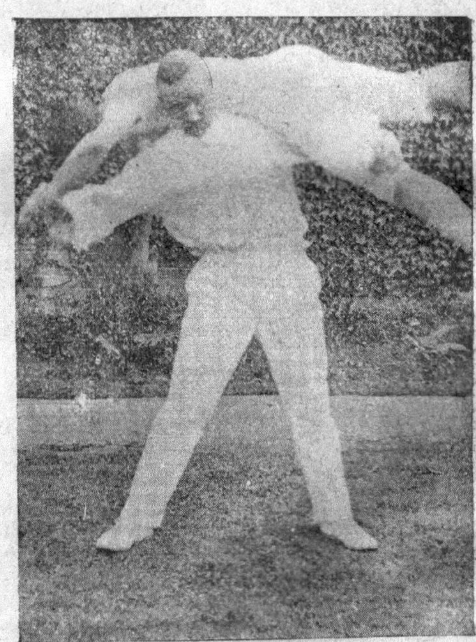

THE WRIST AND THIGH THROW.

Hold tightly and bending forward lay him on his back ; there is no need to do this violently. If it be tried on you, directly your opponent takes hold of your thigh back-heel his advanced leg with your right foot as quickly as possible and you may throw him.

THE ARM SWING.

Grip right wrist in your left hand and placing your right hand on his right arm just above the elbow, so that as you turn it is between your upper arm and side, swing yourself in very quickly to your left, and thus dragging the man with you you can swing him to his back by the hold on the arm alone. This is difficult to stop if done quickly (as it must be), but you should try to grip him round the right thigh from the inside with your free arm and lift and throw.

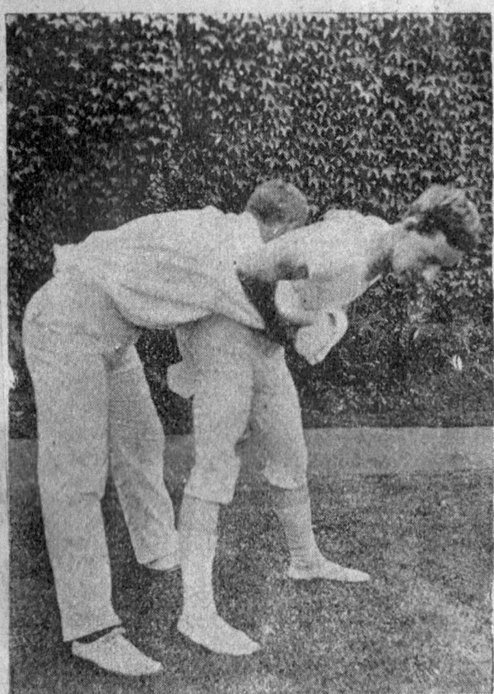

ARM SWING AND STOP.

Never try the arm swing on a man heavier than yourself.

CROSS BUTTOCK.

Seize right wrist with your left hand and right upper arm in your right, turn your side to the man, being somewhat close to him, and strike both his legs from under him with your right leg, swinging him forward at the same time. This opportunity of crossing a man's legs frequently occurs during struggling, although use is but seldom made of it. It is very difficult to stop, and a hard and unlooked-for fall results.

NECK TWIST.

Obtain hold as for buttock, stepping forward then, by a sudden move release the neck and slip the right hand over the shoulder and under the left armpit and hold firmly. The man's head is now pressed against your right side, release the right wrist and strengthen the hold with your left arm brought under his chest and clasping hands or wrist, then with a strong twist to the right you can twist the man to the ground, as the neck cannot withstand the strain thrown on it

It sometimes happens that you are able to get hold of both your opponent's thighs, if you can you are able to tumble him backwards easily. To stop this he should withdraw his legs as far as possible and may try the counter by leaning over and grasping you round the loins.

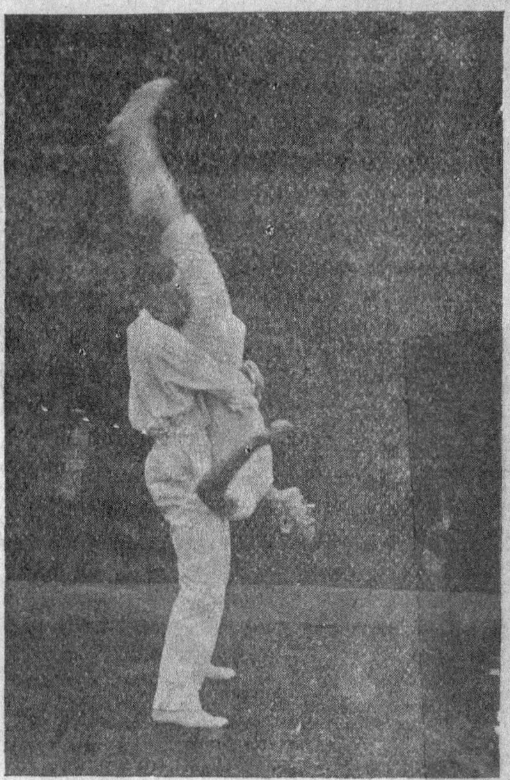

No. 11.—COUNTER TO BOTH THIGHS HOLD.

If he be strong enough he can now lift you, turning you heels over head, and swing you to his shoulders, from which position he may throw you by swinging you again heels over head to his left side (if you be on his right shoulder) to your back. This is a complicated move but wonderfully effective. It should never be attempted, however, without personal instruction, and unless a fair amount of strength be possessed, otherwise an accident may easily occur. There is nothing brutal about it in the least, but it must be thoroughly understood, or let alone. If you are grasped by your opponent round the body after he has withdrawn his legs, you may get in a splendid counter stroke, if you act instantly. Seize both his elbows and rise up suddenly, and you will throw him a complete somersault over your back (see illustration on page 14).

The foregoing are some of the best throws obtainable in this style, but there are, of course, many others to be used as circumstances or necessity require.

When the men come to the ground, and one attempts to turn the other to his back, it is best for him to get in the half-Nelson first. To make this, pass your left hand under the left armpit of your opponent and place it firmly on his neck, from this hold, assisted by the other arm, most of the twists and turns from the ground are made. Take care in ground wrestling—(the half - Nelson may b.

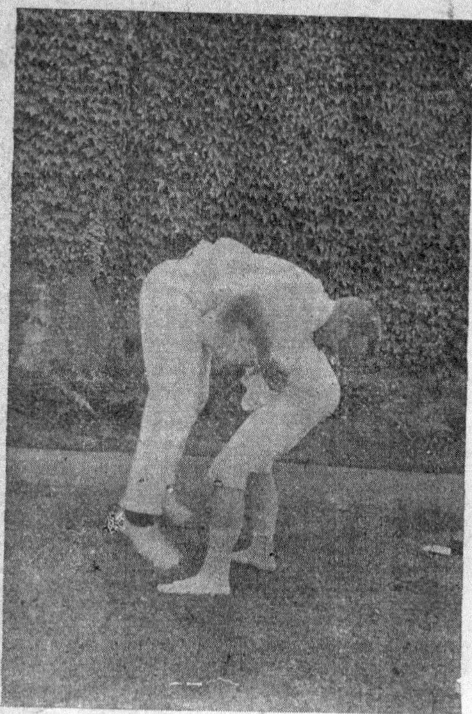

COUNTER TO No. II.

Nelson, but these are not permitted at Amateur contests, where a judge has power to disqualify a man whom he thinks is using undue violence in order to secure a fall.

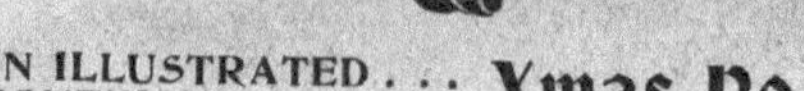

Editorial Notes.

I HAVE very little space wherein to say a lot I would like to say. Firstly, one or two things promised for this issue are crowded out, and will appear in the next grand Christmas Number. All the same, I would like to hear from any reader who does not agree that this issue of the magazine is the best yet published. You will no doubt remember that I promised to make each future issue more interesting and useful than the preceding month's. But a bigger stride of improvement than ever will be made with the Christmas Number. Below I reproduce the cover design and *the number of pages will be increased to 48* (OR MORE). Among illustrations will be a splendid close back view photo of Mr. Vansittart, also life size photo of the huge nail bent by him, fine photos of Max Milian and Mr. Von Lom (with interview), of London Central Weight Lifting Club, a new pose by Professor Macfadden, photos of a youth before taking up Physical Culture, further photos in three month's time to show development attained, funny caricature sketches of Chest Expander Competition at our office, and others, whilst amongst reading matter will be two readers' replies to Apollo's criticisms of Sandow, "Physical Culture and Mental Culture," "Food as a Cumulative Drug and Poison," a story, "The Strong Man and the Hooligans," new "Tricks and Tests of Muscle," more "Experiences of Physical Culture," a large batch of "Answers to Correspondents," prize competitions, etc., etc. The price will be 3d., and orders should be placed with us or your bookseller or bookstall if you wish to make sure of a copy.

made from either side) not to bring your legs within your opponent's reach, as it his move to seize them, and if he have hold of one of your legs any efforts to turn him are practically useless. In the same way he will endeavour to prevent you getting in the half-Nelson. The usual twist employed is to get at the side of a man and getting in the half-Nelson to push the other arm under the body or under the near and over the far thigh and so lever him over ; or by lying down in a line with the man and passing both arms under his armpit and placing the hands on his back so turn him, keeping his head down by pressing your chest on the back of it. If you can get one arm so fixed draw his opposite hand over to the hip and you can easily turn him. The underneath man should try to imprison an opponent's arm when fixed and rising slightly endeavour to draw him to his shoulders.

I am not at all partial to ground wrestling and in my opinion it is best avoided, if possible, although it must be learned, as so many men rely almost solely on their ground work to defeat an opponent. Remember in ground wrestling to keep the fingers close together when underneath, so as to avoid risk of breakage, and further to seize the first opportunity of regaining the feet, as nothing is more exhausting than struggling on the ground.

There are several throws in use amongst American professional catch-hold wrestlers which depend almost solely on the pain caused to an opponent by their use, such as Strangle, Shoulder Twist, Backhammer and Double

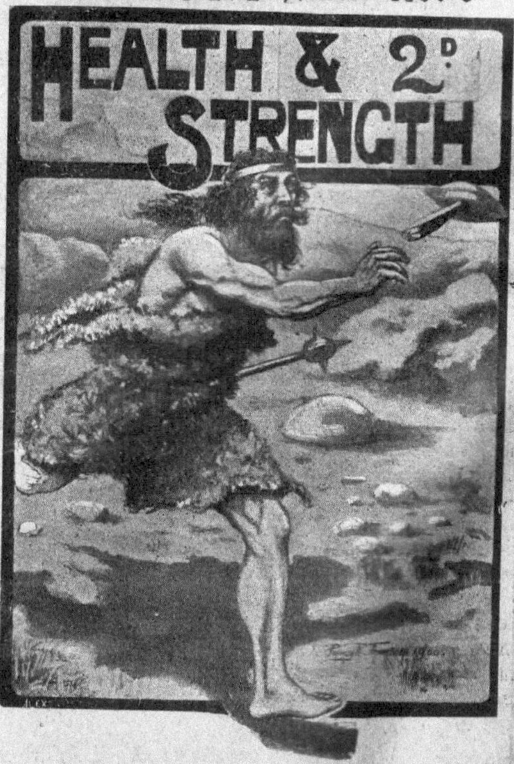

Professor Macfadden's Fasting Experiment.

Seven Days Without Liquid or Solid Food, and Still Strong Enough to Raise 100-lb. Dumb-bell Overhead with One Hand.

Want to be made over new? Want to cure your complaints and feel the returning powers of youth? Want to rid yourself of impurities that clog the system and produce all sorts of diseases? If so, fast from four to thirty days.

Talk about tonics! Why, there is only one tonic in the world that will give you the same appetite, the same joy of youth and life as will the after-results of fasting.

For the last fifteen years I have frequently fasted as a means of aiding in curing threatened illnesses that attack even the most careful in this age of civilized or rather uncivilized dietary.

I have been seriously threatened with pneumonia and numerous other ills of less importance which have quickly succumbed to this effective means of ridding the system of impurities. Though there are now some valuable works on this subject, when I first adopted these theories they were based entirely on my own intelligence and instinct and the knowledge that all animals fasted when ill.

Until this last experiment, which forms the subject of this article, four days was the longest time that it ever became necessary for me to fast, and even then I usually ate an apple or a bite or two of something light each day, thus at no time previous to this last experiment did I fast absolutely.

I have frequently made comments on the value of fasting in this Magazine, and determined to test the effects of an absolute fast of one week on strength and weight. I did not take a particle of nourishment in any form, though drank very freely of pure water.

The first day of the fast I lost five pounds and the next day two pounds, and the loss gradually decreased each day, and on the day was but little over one pound. Altogether in the seven days my total loss of weight was fifteen pounds.

Each day I walked about ten miles, and surprising as it may seem, I felt weaker on the second day of the fast than at any time thereafter.

I always took my walk in the morning immediately on rising and usually felt quite weak at the start. This was, however, entirely a morbid feeling, for after travelling one or two miles it would entirely disappear and I could walk with a strong steady tread, and at the conclusion always felt equal to ten or twenty miles more.

The first four days were the most uncomfortable. I did not seem especially hungry, but I was languid, except for a while after exercise, at which times I always felt strong and energetic.

I attended to my daily duties during the entire fast with the same regularity as usual. My brain seemed especially clear, and mental work actually required less effort than when eating regularly.

Frequently when rising from a seat after a short rest during the first three or four days of the fast, I would feel quite dizzy for a few moments, but this would quickly pass away.

At times difficulty was experienced in inducing sleep. The gnawing sensation in my stomach would not cease, though a plentiful supply of cool pure water seemed of great advantage, and was of valuable assistance in wooing slumber.

The sixth and seventh days of the fast were really by far the most comfortable. I felt that it would require but little effort to continue on for three or four weeks, but the object of the fast was accomplished and I was not at all anxious to continue it further.

The most important feature in lessening the effects of fasting is to keep the mind employed so it will not be continually referring to the desire for food.

The only time there was the slightest danger of my giving way to my appetite was on the fourth day. At this particular time I mention, there was nothing of importance for me to do, and after conversing a short time with some friends, I went out with the distinct intention of patronising the nearest restaurant.

After walking a block or two and giving the matter serious consideration, I determined not to break the fast, and instead of the restaurant, I went to the gymnasium and spent thirty minutes in vigorous exercise, and I felt much better, and all thoughts of giving up the fast were abandoned.

The comparison photographs show how the body wasted away during the fast. The face thinned especially and the eyes sunk considerably.

But the astounding fact in connection with the fast was the strength possessed on the seventh day. The average person imagines that he becomes weak even after missing a meal, and a fast of one day is supposed to take away all strength. There was never greater error.

On the fourth day of the fast after testing my strength, I concluded to use a 50-lb. dumbbell in illustrating my strength on the seventh day of the fast.

Well, the seventh day came at last, though I must confess the week seemed rather long. I visited the gymnasium after my walk with the intention of leaving instructions that the 50-lb. dumb-bell be sent around to the photograph gallery. On arriving there I felt so strong that I concluded to test my strength. I thought that may be I might be able to raise without difficulty a heavier dumb-bell than 50-lbs.

I raised the 50-lb. dumb-bell over my head a number of times without the slightest difficulty. It did not seem heavier than when at my usual weight. I tried the 60-lb. bell, then the 70-lb., and 85-lb. with similar results, and immediately left instructions to send the 100-lb. bell over to the photograph gallery as I felt that my strength was equal to raising it.

I know full well that my readers will be amazed at these feats of strength performed after this long fast, and no one could be more amazed than I, for as stated before I was under the impression that to raise a 50-lb. bell over head with one hand after a fast of this character would really be something worth boasting about, and to say that I was astounded at my strength under the circumstances is putting it very mildly.

The 100-lb. dumb-bell was sent to the gallery, and Sarony's employees who saw and photographed the feats will vouch for the statements made and the illustrations shown. I had to raise the 100-lb. dumb-bell twice before a proper negative could be made of the feat.

The second feat of raising a 200-lb. man, as shown in the photographs, was not easy, as anyone will discover on trial, and it would be well to remember that I never at any time in my athletic career believed in using heavy weights, and had not attempted to raise a 100-lb. dumb-bell off the floor for at least two years before these feats were performed.

While in active practice in general athletic work a number of years ago, I could raise a 100-lb. bell eleven times at arm's length over head with one arm, but at this time I frequently handled heavy weights. As I have taken no heavy exercise for a number of years, more than a slight effort would be required to raise this heavy dumb-bell, even when my weight was at its usual standard. A lesson is taught with unquestionable clearness by this experiment.

The American [and English.—The Ed.] people are actually eating themselves into their graves. Ninety-nine out of every hundred take from five to fifty years from the length of their lives by stuffing their stomachs. They eat, not to nourish the body, but merely for the pleasure of gourmandizing. The result is that from two to five times as much food passes through the alimentary canal than is necessary to maintain weight and strength, and mind and body are actually weakened by the strenuous efforts made by the system in endeavouring to rid itself of this excessive amount of food.

Though I thoroughly believe that anyone can be benefitted by intelligent fasting at times, let me here warn each faster against the serious injury that will result from over-eating after a fast. Begin to eat very slowly. All the benefit of your abstinence will be lost if this advice is not given due attention.

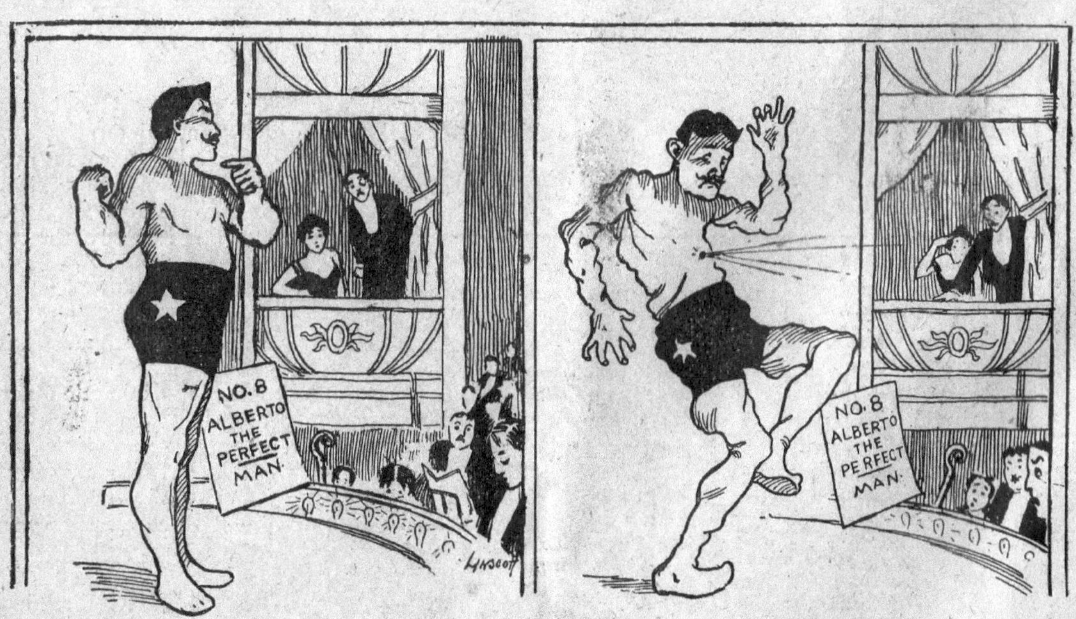

TAKING THE WIND OUT OF HIS SAILS.

"THE BEST TONIC I HAVE EVER COME ACROSS."

" . . . . . Some time ago I purchased a Macfadden MassageRoller from you on approval. Well, as you have not received it back again, you will have assumed, and rightly too, that I am perfectly satisfied, if not delighted, with it.

And so, indeed, I am. It is about the best tonic I have ever come across. The refreshment and energy one feels after five or ten minutes' use is simply astonishing.

However, it is not the purpose of this letter to eulogise your splendid invention, although I can well understand the satisfaction that is yours on receiving so glowing an opinion " (*Here our correspondent's letter goes on to other matters*).

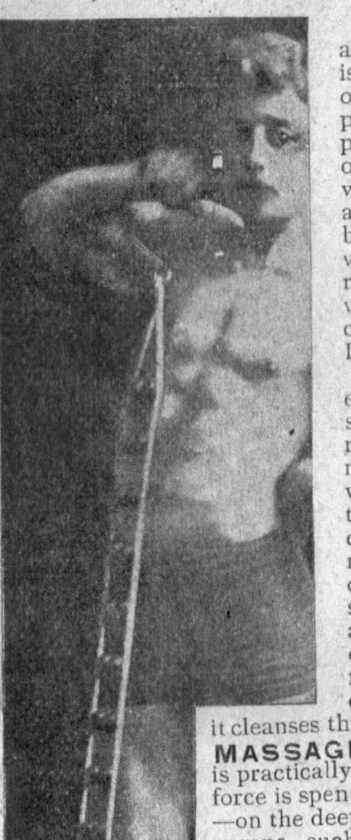

The highest standard of development is impossible without Massage. It plays an important part in the training of professional, as well as amateur, athletes, including boxers, runners, wrestlers, jumpers, rovers, &c., and was used by the ancient Greeks and Romans.

Feats of unusual endurance are possible only as the result of the elimination of poisonous waste from the system, and it is such elimination that makes soldiers and others "fit." Massage does quickly and easily what otherwise takes months or years of exercise to do, viz., it cleanses the system. With the **MASSAGE-ROLLER** there is practically no friction, and the force is spent where it should be —on the deeper structures and organs, such as the Stomach, Liver and Intestines, on Muscles and Nerves. The quickly intermitting pressure from the balls drives along rapidly and vigourously the blood, and thus hastens those cell changes on which life and health depend.

Those who have purchased one of our Massage-Rollers say they would not take five or ten times its cost could they not get another. You cannot afford not to give it a trial, and this we shall be pleased to allow, as we will promptly refund your money if at the end of a week's practical trial you are not of the same opinion.

A 122-page handsomely illustrated book "The Natural Prevention and Cure of Disease," giving instructions in detail for treating all sorts of diseases, accompanies each machine (excepting 3/6 pattern) *free.* Send for *one now.* It costs you nothing to try it. Book alone 2/2 post free.

PRICES—3/6 (Non-stretching), **6/6** (Stretching), or **10/6** (Stretching and Cork Handles). Postage 5d. extra.

H ealth & Strength Co.. 73, Farringdon St,, E.C.

Dr, GEORGE HORATIO JONES,
THE OLD ESTABLISHED SURGEON DENTIST, OF
57, Great Russell Street
(*Directly facing the British Museum*), *may be consulted daily, as usual, for the*
Best English and American Dentistry,
Moderate Fees. Extension of Premises, Great Russell Mansions next door. See name under "Dentists," Post Office Directory.

Diet to be Determined by Exercise.

HENRY A. GRIFFIN, M.D., in an article on "Foods," in the *Independent*, says:—

"Emphasis must be laid upon an evil which is far too prevalent, and of which investigators and writers upon dietetics are constantly urging abatement. This is the tendency to overeat. It is no easy thing perhaps to sit before a table groaning with good things and surrounded by those who, like ourselves, enjoy them, and then to practice moderation ; but while over-indulgence may go unpunished for a time, sooner or later, if food be taken in excess of

always be provided for, and hence a 'hearty appetite' in childhood is—within limits—a thing to be encouraged.

"In full growth, however, of necessity the food is taken only to repair waste, and the amount to be taken can readily be determined by each individual. In old age the require-ment for food is still less, for with advancing years there is less exercise. A small amount of food will therefore suffice to maintain the nutrition of the aged, though, owing to the digestive enfeeblement of old age, that little

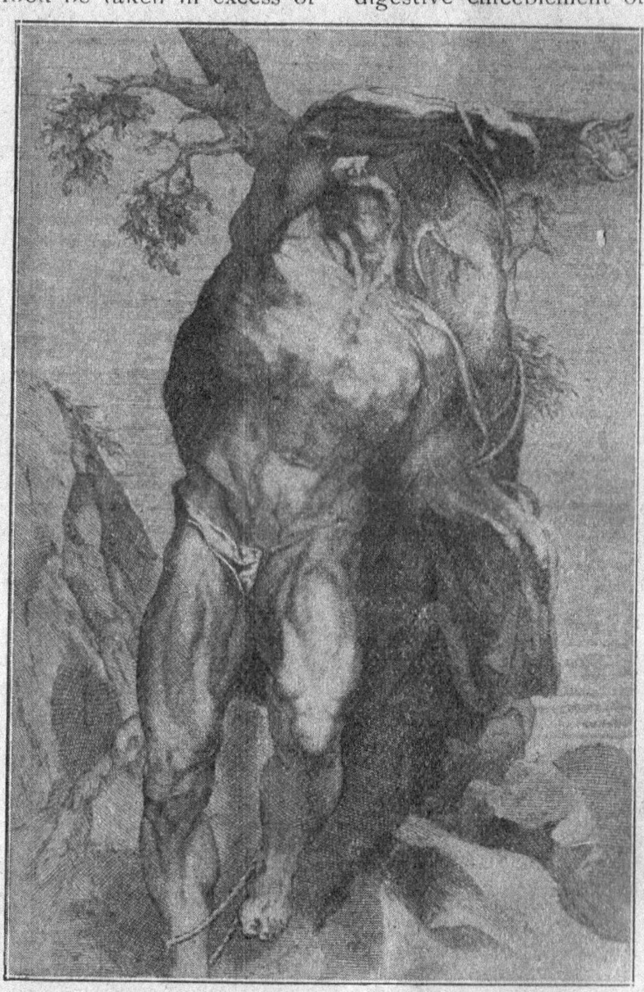

PROMETHEUS BOUND.

the demands of the body and purely at the in-stigation of the appetite, a day of retribution will come when, in bilious misery, if no worse, we recognise that enough is sufficient.

"How much each should eat will be a matter for each to determine by experience. The young properly eat more in proportion to their size than those of full growth, because like all young animals they are more active, and therefore have more waste to repair. Further than that, however, in them the re-pair of waste is not sufficient, for growth must

should be simple, nourishing, and susceptible of easy digestion.

"Diet should wait on exercise ; for, mani-festly, if food is taken to provide the means for vital powers shown in motion, and little motion is required, then little food should be used, and that of the least hearty kinds, else a harmful accumulation. To feed the labourer and the student alike would be folly ; for the tissue waste of the former is great, while that of the sedentary liver is very small indeed ; therefore the latter requires much less food than the former.

What the Microscope Reveals !

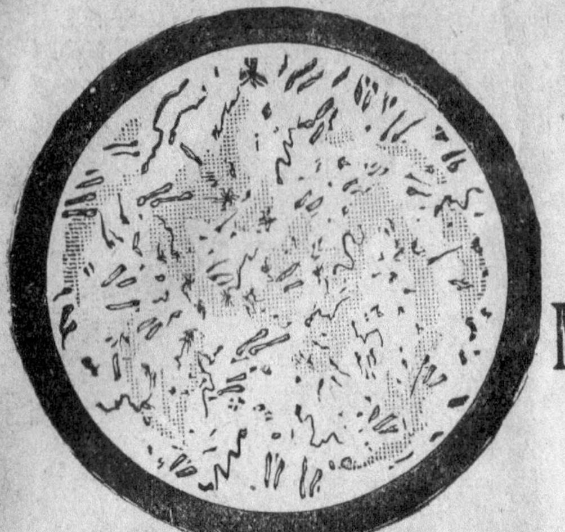

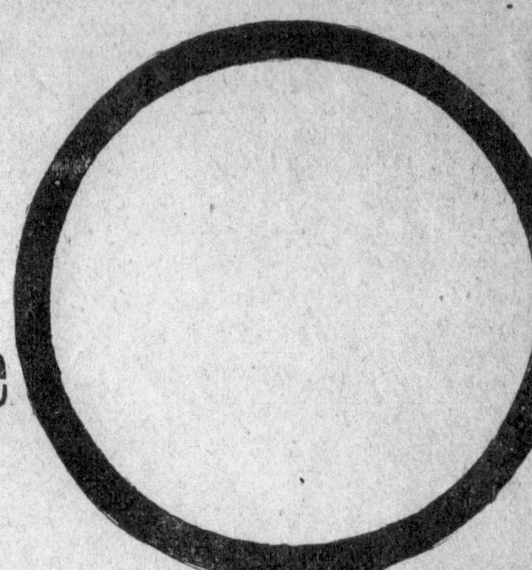

Which Will You Drink ?

Thousands of cities, towns, and villages in the United Kingdom are daily emptying their sewerage, filth, slops, decayed animal and vegetable matter into our rivers, lakes and streams. It is little cause for wonder then, considering the amount of water we each consume in one form or another that we have a race of people, prematurely aged, nervous, wrinkled, rheumatic and dyspeptic, when the seeds of ill-health are sown daily. It makes no difference where you live, in crowded city or on a farm, you cannot be sure of pure water. You may filter your water, but the germs of disease are still there. Dr. Andrew Wilson recently stated that you might as well drink unfiltered water in so far as the power of an ordinary filter to remove disease germs from water is concerned. Distillation is the only method of purifying the water we drink, and this can only be done effectually and economically by means of

The Puritan PURE WATER Still,

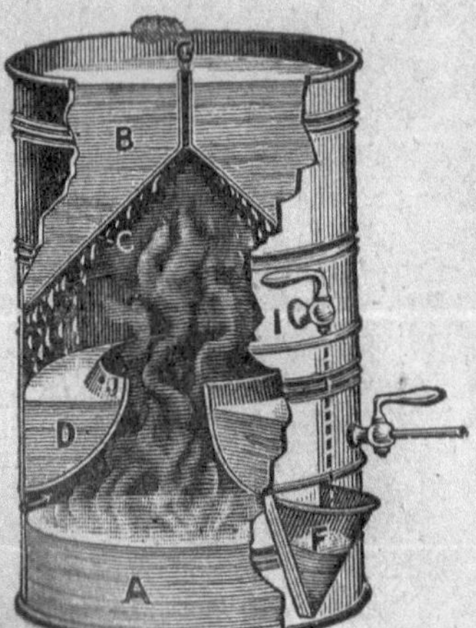

Which will produce from the foulest liquid a beautiful supply of soft, sparkling water, clear to the eye, and free from mud, lime, salts or microbes. Puritan distilled water is simply pure steam, condensed, aërated and revitalized.

DR. ANDREW WILSON, the eminent physician, in an article on "The Typhoid Fever Season" in *Daily Mail* of 18th September says: "If you ensure that you drink pure water you will go far to escape infection from abroad. My advice to my readers is

NEVER DRINK ORDINARY WATER.

Dr. R. N. Tooker, Chicago, writes:—"For flushing the kidneys, stimulating the sluggish liver, eliminating waste matter from the system, indeed for all affections which medicinal waters are believed to be efficacious, pure distilled water urnishes the long sought desideratum."

25/- Postage 9d. extra.

Recommended by the Editor of "HEALTH AND STRENGTH."

Send for Illustrated "P" Pamphlet, post free, or call and Inspect the Still in operation.

AGENTS WANTED.

The Gem Supplies Co., 6, Bishop's Court near P.O.)
Chancery Lane, London, E.C.

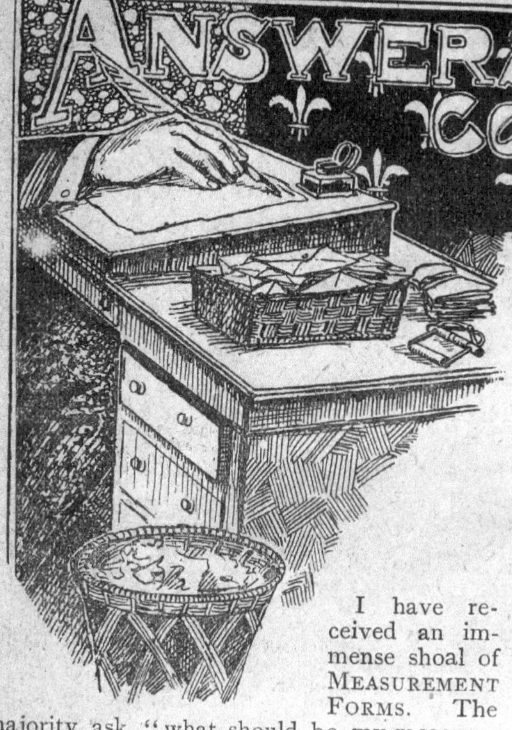

I have received an immense shoal of MEASUREMENT FORMS. The majority ask "what should be my measurements?" and I now give a collective answer to all such enquiries—present and future—in the form of a table, showing (approximately) the highest standard (not average) weights and measurements of adults (age 20 to 30) of different heights. The figures do not represent a hard and fast guide. A fleshy man, for instance, stands a much better chance of equalling these figures than a small-boned and slightly-built man. After all, quality and strength of muscle is a truer test of health and strength than mere bulk:—

Height.	Weight.	Chest.	Upper-arm.	Fore-arm.	Waist.	Thigh.
5ft. 1in.	8st. 6lbs	34 in.	11½in.	9 in.	29½in.	16 in.
5 ,, 2 ,,	8 ,, 13 ,,	35·1	12 ,,	9½ ,,	30 ,,	17 ,,
5 ,, 3 ,,	9 ,, 4 ,,	35·7	12½ ,,	10 ,,	30½ ,,	18 ,,
5 ,, 4 ,,	9 ,, 11 ,,	36·2	13 ,,	10½ ,,	31 ,,	19 ,,
5 ,, 5 ,,	10 ,, 1 ,,	36·7	13½ ,,	10⅞ ,,	31½ ,,	20 ,,
5 ,, 6 ,,	10 ,, 5 ,,	37·5	14 ,,	11 ,,	32 ,,	21 ,,
5 ,, 7 ,,	10 ,, 7 ,,	38·1	14½ ,,	11½ ,,	32½ ,,	22 ,,
5 ,, 8 ,,	10 ,, 12 ,,	38·5	15 ,,	11⅛ ,,	33 ,,	23 ,,
5 ,, 9 ,,	11 ,, 4 ,,	39·1	15½ ,,	12 ,,	33½ ,,	24 ,,
5 ,, 10 ,,	11 ,, 11 ,,	39·6	16 ,,	12½ ,,	34 ,,	25 ,,
5 ,, 11 ,,	12 ,, 2 ,,	40·2	16½ ,,	12⅞ ,,	34½ ,,	26 ,,
6 feet.	12 ,, 7 ,,	41·0	17 ,,	13 ,,	35 ,,	27 ,,

NOTE.—The fractions in the Chest Measurements are ⅒ths. The girth of the Neck and Calf should be about the same as the Upper-arm.

Excema? R. S. CLAPTON.—Blood needs purifying by regular exercise, suitable dietary and plenty of fresh air. Don't overeat. Two meals a day would be better than three. Drop pigmeat and rich dishes, sauces and irritative condiments. Eat plenty of vegetables (especially green stuff) and fruit

Is it possible to increase height 1-in.? A NEW READER, ROCHDALE.—Enquirer is afraid if he increases chest measurement he will spoil his chance of increasing height. He is 5-ft. 8-in. with 33-in. chest, and it seems to me that chest increase is more necessary than increase of height. Anyway, an increase of chest will help to increase height—not retard it.

Blackheads and Indigestion? E. W. H., DUBLIN.—Only 18 and afflicted with indigestion. See answer to "R. S., CLAPTON."

Pigeon chest. T. A. P., PLAISTOW.—You need exercises for chest expansion. Dumb-bells will not help you so well as a Chest Expander or Exerciser. Shall be pleased to recommend suitable exercises if you will use either.

Indigestion, chronic sore throat, general debility, catarrh of right lung? CONSTANT READER, LONDON.—Yours is a bad case for one only 20 years. Your clerical occupation should be thrown up for an outdoor life with plenty of exercise, or I fear you will never be strong and healthy.

Intense desire to go to sleep in daytime, especially after mid-day dinner? F. R., GRAYS, ESSEX.— Your liver seems inactive. Exercise regularly and eat only twice per day, at noon and late dinner. If hungry in morning eat a little fruit in season, or dried fruits like raisins, figs and dates.

Blushing? Is it proper to plunge into cold water after exercise? U. G., GLASGOW.—Blushing is a common complaint at your age, and you will grow out of it. Cold water will not hurt you if your heart is not weak. If it causes your heart to beat too strongly and quickly it would be better to use lukewarm water.

Exercise to increase height? At what age does a youth cease to grow? J. J., MANOR PARK, E.—All round exercise, sleep, breathing and stretching movements of all kinds. Height and growth ceases from 18 to 21. Bulk growth 45 to 55.

Where can PROFESSOR MACFADDEN'S *book,* "Natural Cure of Disease," *etc., etc., be obtained?* C. M., BERTH, AYRSHIRE.—From HEALTH & STRENGTH Co., price 2/-, 2/2 post free, with coupon exchangeable for same amount.

[*A large number of "Answers" are crowded out.*]

The
Athlete's Conquest;

The Romance of an Athlete.

(REVISED).

By BERNARR A. MACFADDEN.

INTRODUCTION.—This highly interesting story commenced in the April issue, and the story in book form will be sent post free for 1/2. The opening of the story relates how HARRY MOORE, a strong, athletic, well-made young man, with a good income, a fine business, had everything necessary to make him happy—except a wife. HARRY MOORE gives us his ideal of a wife—and the story goes on to describe his meeting such a life companion. The story then takes us back five years to a period when our hero was on the point of breaking up as the result of the close confinement of city employment, and goes on to introduce the reader to an interview between HARRY MOORE and an enlightened physican, who holds out a most hopeful prospect. The story goes on to show the nature of the doctor's advice and its happy result, and the hero's thoughts regarding an ideal wife, and his quest for such a life companion.

CHAPTER VIII.—(Continued.)

" Have I forgotten what I suffered? Have I forgotten that there are thousands, yes millions, of young girls and women suffering to-day as I did? Their suffering will last all through life —mine was of short duration, for, by accident, I acquired the proper knowledge of the laws of life. Shall I forget all my suffering sisters and live for my own enjoyment? No! A thousand times No," she cried vehemently.

" I feel that I have a duty to perform," she continued to herself, "I feel that my physical power and beauty were given me for a purpose, and that purpose was to assist in the dissemination of that knowledge which enabled me to obtain this great boon to womankind. I have the power to make every girl, every young woman more beautiful, more healthy, and to-night, yes, even to night, I was about to renounce all.

" I have sent him away, and he shall not return with my consent," she said, half aloud.

She seated herself at the desk and again began to read her lecture.

"Yes!" she read, "the time is not far distant when girls will grow into true womanhood. When they will be the pride and glory of civilization ; when health and beauty will be the rule and not the exception, as it is to-day ; when every young woman will understand the true laws of life, and mock modesty —another name for degraded ignorance and impurity of the mind—will be of the past ; when happiness will be seen on every side : when girls can indulge in health-giving games without criticism, and the true standard of beauty will have buried the corset so deep that its resurrection will be impossible."

She read on and on, page after page. Her features betrayed the great intensity of her feelings, as the written thoughts were conveyed to her mind.

As she put down the manuscript an expression of peace and content was in her eyes, sitting there with clasped hands. " What a power I possess! How glorious to be able to work in such a cause," she said, half aloud, with emotion in her voice.

"He will forgive me, I know. I could' never accomplish this great work if I were married. It might be possible, but I suppose he views marriage from a conventional standpoint, and the duties of a wife and mother would be imposed on me, seriously impairing my usefulness in this great work ; later I may change my opinions, but now the sun shines brightly on my pathway, and it is not from the light of a happy marriage."

———

What were Harry's feelings when he quitted Edith's presence so suddenly? What had caused him to make such a rash proposal? He saw that she was intensely interested in her proposed work. In praising her purpose, his own words thrilled him—moved him so that he formed a noble purpose. He would leave her to follow the bent of her aspirations without his interference. For a moment he felt ashamed for trying to marry her—she seemed so much above him. Why should he interfere with her purpose, especially when of such a worthy nature?

With these self-sacrificing thoughts in his mind, he concluded to risk all. If she seriously desired him to leave her presence for ever, he would obey her wish.

For a moment, as she hesitated, he felt encouraged. Even when she said he should go, he did not lose hope.

"After all," he thought, "she may return my love." But when she said so emphatically, "Yes, you must go," he feared his doom was sealed. But even then a ray of hope remained.

"Why does she turn away from me?" he thought, and he asked her to look up into his eyes. But her only answer was to beg him to go, and it was too much.

He thought that she so hated to cause him pain that it made her suffer. He called himself a brute, and braced himself for the few final words he said in parting.

He went down the stone steps with all hope for happiness left behind. In that moment the nobleness of that man's character, and his great, magnanimous love for Edith were shown

TURKISH BATHS AT HOME.

Everybody has known something of the value of Turkish baths, but only a few could afford them Those few kept well—kept mind and body up to the highest vigour. The rest let impurities accumulate; and often the end was a wreck. Then the victim goes to a sanitarium or elsewhere to let Turkish baths cure what they might have prevented.

With a **CENTURY FOLDING CABINET** you can now take Turkish baths at home at a cost of 1½d. per bath. You can keep well and cure yourself, so far as Turkish baths can do it. In most ills nothing can do more. Nobody is so poor nor so remote that he cannot enjoy the luxury of the Roman bath. Nobody can keep clean or vigorous or maintain a clear complexion without it.

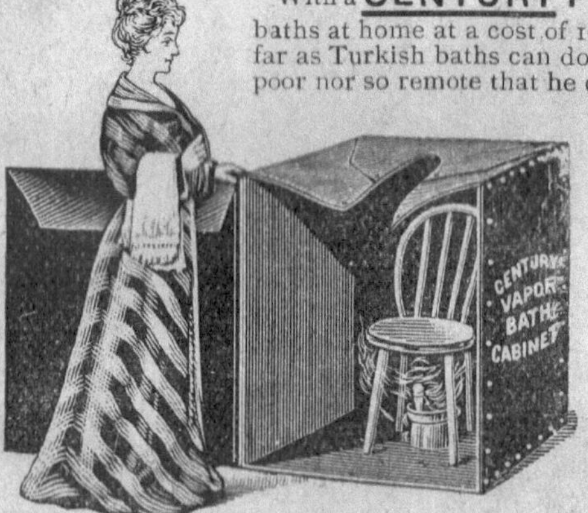

Some kind of blood poisoning is the cause of nearly all ill-health. A poisonous acid in the blood causes rheumatism. Other poisons wreck the nerves. Nicotine weakens the smoker's heart. Blood impurity shows in a thousand ways, and unless one forces the poison out through the pores, it must go through the kidneys, and the tax breaks the kidneys down.

The quick, powerful, certain way to remove these impurities is by forcing them out through the pores. Nobody can doubt that.

Add to this the luxury, the comforting, sleep-bringing, vim-producing qualities. Add cleanliness and clearness of complexion. Add their service in stopping all colds at once. The pleasure of life may be doubled and sickness reduced more than half by the habit of Turkish Bathing.

PRICE complete with Spirit Heater & Vaporizer

25/- to 70/-

Free 35 Formulas for Medicated Baths.

THE CENTURY THERMAL BATH CABINET.

Is guaranteed to be the best on the market. It is built on a steel frame with Hygienic Waterproof Cloth and *folds up like a screen into 2-inch space, weight 20-lbs*. The top consists of four flaps or curtains and admits of **four distinct temperatures.** We sell on 15 days' trial (to be returned if not as represented).

The **Face Steamer** used with Cabinet gives beautiful complexion and cures Colds, Bronchitis, Asthma. **Sample of Goods,** and Valuable Book, sent **free** on receipt of Address. **Write** to-day.

AGENTS WANTED. *Exclusive Rights.*

H.D., Century Thermal Bath Cabinet, Ltd. (Dept. 83), 203. & 205, Regent St., London, W.

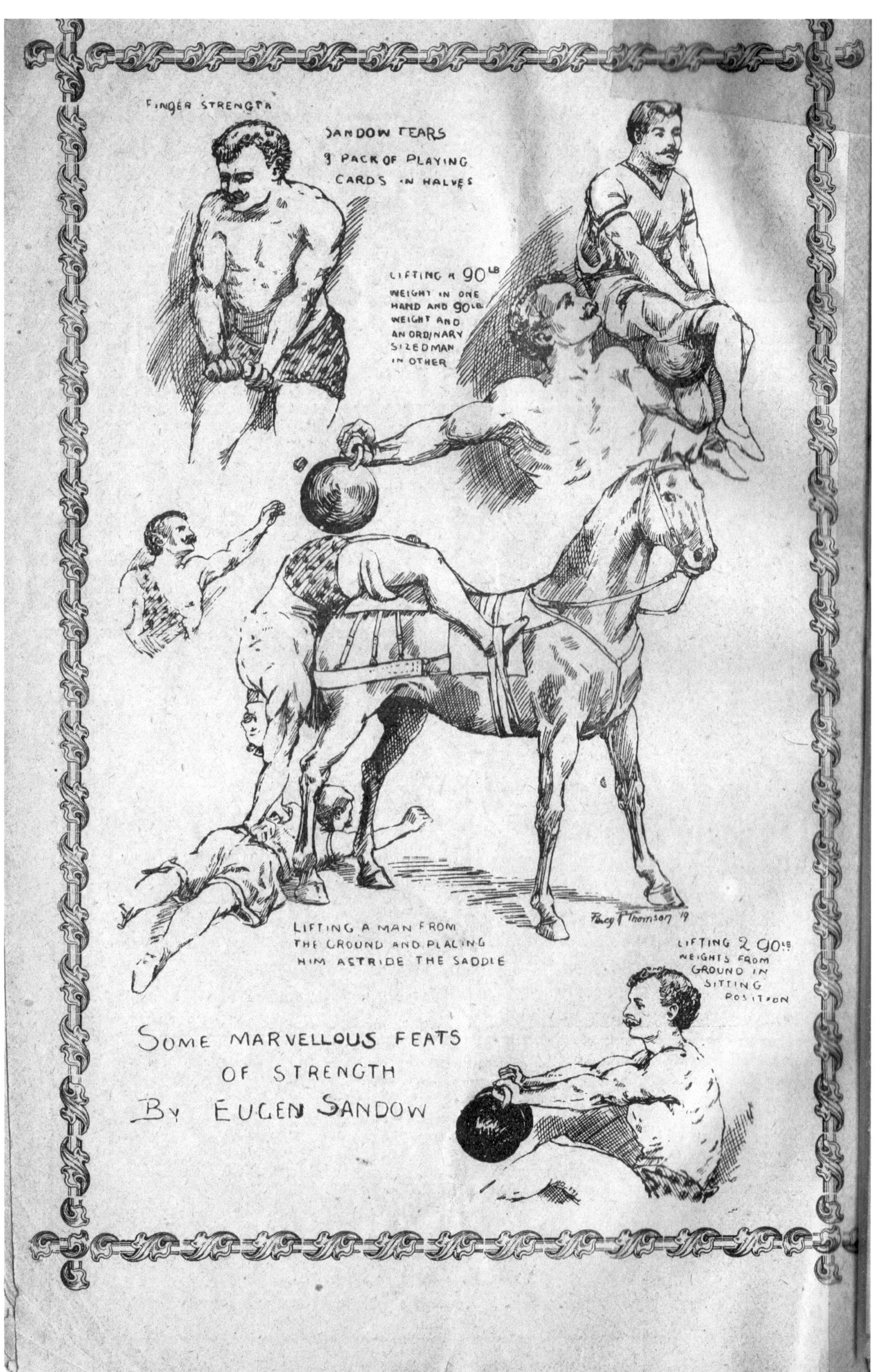

FINGER STRENGTH
SANDOW TEARS A PACK OF PLAYING CARDS IN HALVES
LIFTING A 90 LB WEIGHT IN ONE HAND AND 90 LB WEIGHT AND AN ORDINARY SIZED MAN IN OTHER
LIFTING A MAN FROM THE GROUND AND PLACING HIM ASTRIDE THE SADDLE
LIFTING 2 90 LB WEIGHTS FROM GROUND IN SITTING POSITION
Percy T Thomson 19
SOME MARVELLOUS FEATS OF STRENGTH
BY EUGEN SANDOW

with remarkable clearness. He had his faults like all men, but there were moments when his imagination carried him into the upper realm, and his last thought was for himself. There are men, there are women, with such natures. In the ordinary vocation of life they are as others; but when something of great importance arises, when it becomes necessary to risk life or make great sacrifices, they spring forward with alacrity.

How we love this trait, so seldom seen in this day of selfishness and race for gain. Rushing, crushing, crowding, down the stream of life they go, each one striving to be uppermost. If, in the efforts to gain the desired position, one forces a human being under the water of life's stream, it makes no difference. "It's all in the game, you know," he will grin and say to himself. It is money, money, money, everywhere!

Harry walked towards his home with his face drawn and rigid. A miserable, glaring light was in his eyes. So tightly had he clenched his hands that his finger-nails brought blood. He believed that he could win Edith's love if he persisted in his attentions. But in his present mood he was willing to sacrifice his chances because she seemed to conscientiously desire him to do so. He had offered to make this sacrifice and she had accepted, and he would disturb her no more.

(*To be continued.*)

[Complete in book form with portrait of hero, price 1/-, or 1/2 post free,]

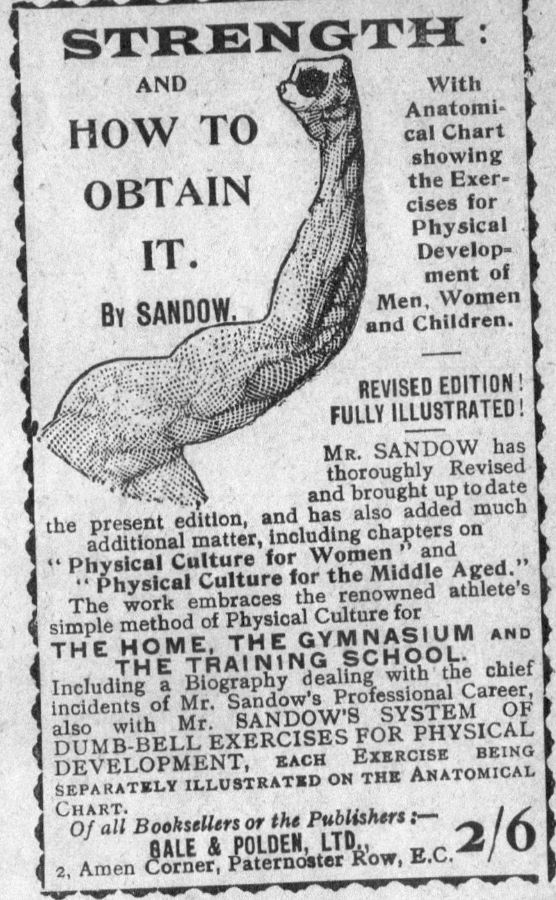

REVISED EDITION! FULLY ILLUSTRATED!

Mr. SANDOW has thoroughly Revised and brought up to date the present edition, and has also added much additional matter, including chapters on "Physical Culture for Women" and "Physical Culture for the Middle Aged." The work embraces the renowned athlete's simple method of Physical Culture for THE HOME, THE GYMNASIUM AND THE TRAINING SCHOOL. Including a Biography dealing with the chief incidents of Mr. Sandow's Professional Career, also with Mr. SANDOW'S SYSTEM OF DUMB-BELL EXERCISES FOR PHYSICAL DEVELOPMENT, EACH EXERCISE BEING SEPARATELY ILLUSTRATED ON THE ANATOMICAL CHART.

Of all Booksellers or the Publishers:— GALE & POLDEN, LTD., 2, Amen Corner, Paternoster Row, E.C. 2/6

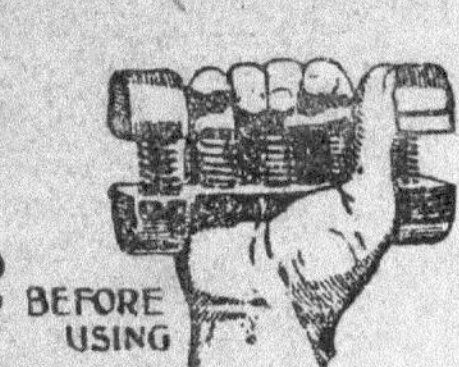

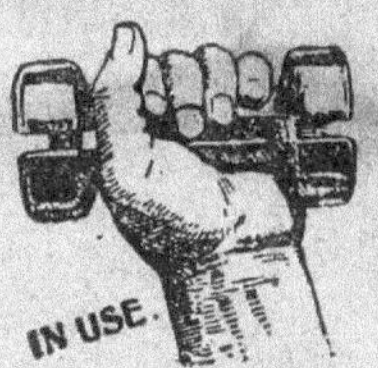

Sandow's Latest

PATENT
SPRING-GRIP DUMB-BELLS

The Greatest Invention of the Age for Producing Perfect Health, Strength and Increased and Proportionate Development.

The Army use them   The Navy use them.   The London Fire Brigade use them.   Doctors use them.   Travellers use them.   Ladies use them.   City Men use them. Children use them.   Hospitals use them.   Cricketers use them.   Footballers use them.   Athletes use them. Gymnasts use them.   Everybody should use them.
SANDOW USES THEM.

You should use the Spring-grip Dumb-bell because:—

1.—Exercise is useless without will-power. The grip on the dumb-bell compels the use of will-power.
2.—There is no danger of any strain on the heart.
3.—The heaviest Spring-Grip Dumb-bell weighs only about 3 lbs. The Ladies' and Youths' Bells weigh only about 2 lbs. ; the Boys' and Girls' Bells about 1 lb. ; the Children's about ¾ lb.
4.—An Athlete can do more with these bells than any other whatsoever.
5.—A child can use them.
6.—They last a life time, and one does not require to be continually purchasing heavier bells
7.—As one's development increases, pace can be kept with it by adjusting the springs.
8.—They prevent swing and jerk getting into the work
9.—They are light, and may easily be carried anywhere.
10—SANDOW USES THEM.

Strengthens and Developes the Whole Human Frame, Gives Health, Strength, and Will-Power.

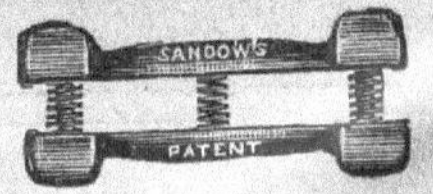

	Nickel Plated with Illustrated Chart, specially prepared by Eugen Sandow, in box complete		
Children			5/-
Girls'	do.	do.	7/6
Boys'	do.	do.	7/6
Ladies'	do.	do.	10/6
Youths'	do.	do.	10/6
Gentlemen	do.	do.	12/6
do.	*In Black Enamel with Illustrated Chart by Eugen Sandow*		7/6

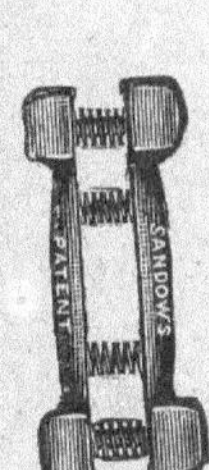

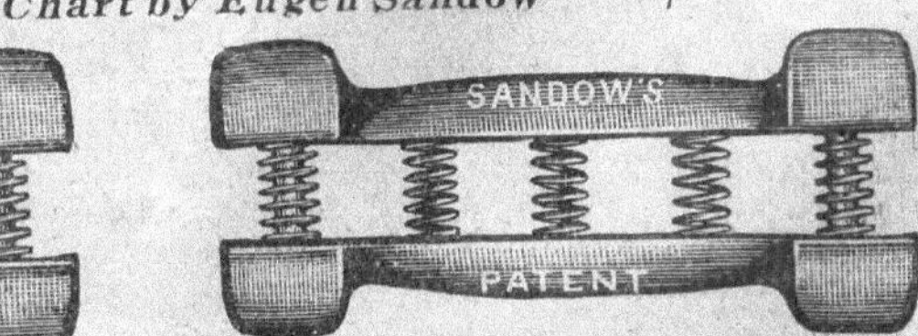

The Dumb-bells showing only 2 Springs in Use.

The Dumb-bells showing all 5 Springs in Use.

THE PUBLIC ARE WARNED AGAINST BUYING SPURIOUS IMITATIONS.

To be had of all Dealers or direct from the Manufacturers :

Sandow's Physical Appliance Co.,
Sandow Hall, Victoria Embankment, London, W.C.

SANDOW'S

2/6

INSTRUCTION BY POST.

Figure showing pupils how to take their own measurements.

In response to numerous enquiries from those who cannot attend his Schools of Physical Culture, Mr. Sandow has pleasure in announcing that he has made arrangements for prescribing courses of Physical Culture at home suited to the individual needs of each pupil. Particulars are given below.

Measurement Form.

Money enclosed ......

Course desired ....

DATE..........................19

NAME ....

ADDRESS ....

PARTICULARS.

Heart, condition of ....

Lungs, condition of ....

Nature of illness, if any.......................... How long ago? ....

Digestion condition of. .... Physical peculiarity, if any ....

Age...... .... Occupation... ....

Athletics, if any.......................... How long ago? ....

Have you "Strength and How to obtain it?" .... Have you "Grip" Dumb-Bell? ....

Have you a Developer? .... Reference No.......................... of last Course.

NECK.	CHEST CONTRACT'D.	CHEST EXPANDED.	UPPER RIGHT ARM.	UPPER LEFT ARM.	FOREARM RIGHT.	FOREARM LEFT.	WAIST.

THIGH RIGHT.	THIGH LEFT.	CALF RIGHT.	CALF LEFT.	HEIGHT.	WEIGHT.

NOTICE.—Fill up this Form, or a similar one, and forward, together with Postal Order, to **EUGEN SANDOW** Instruction Department, Sandow Hall, Savoy Corner, Victoria Embankment. **W.C.**, and you will receive a Complete Course of Instruction lasting for any required period, prescribing exercises with any apparatus the pupil possesses.

Mark Envelope "INSTRUCTION" in Corner.

Sandow's Large Dumb-bell Chart given free with each first course, usual price, 1s. 6d.

1 **Month's Course, 2s. 6d.; 3 Months', 7s.; 6 Months', 12s. 6d.; 12 Months', £1 1s.**
A Conjoint Course, lasting for one month, and consisting of Grip Dumb-Bell Exercises, together with Selected Exercises on Developer and Expander, will be given for **5s.**

SANDOW'S World-wide Competition, 10 GOLD, 10 SILVER, and 50 BRONZE MEDALS offered to those who show the best results from 3 Months' Postal Instruction

☛ FOR ALL PARTICULARS APPLY TO SANDOW HALL. ☚

Dumb-Bells of every description, and all appliances for the study of Physical Culture may be obtained on application to Sandow Hall. Forwarded to any part of the World.

EUGEN SANDOW, Instruction Dept., Crown & Sceptre Court, 32, St. James's St., London, S.W.

PETERSFIELD'S TRAINING CODE.

WITH ADVANCED SERIES.

Absolutely the Finest Home Training on the Market.

You may above double your strength in **3 months** by following the easy graduated course laid down **ten minutes** each day.

It has splendid new methods and requires neither special nor expensive apparatus.

It does what it says, and

"PETERSFIELD"

The Amateur Champion Strong Man declares two inches increase of Biceps nothing extraordinary by his easy graduated scale.

Send for a Copy at once.

Second Edition now in the Press.

Money gladly refunded if not satisfied in one week.

POST FREE 1/-

PETERSFIELD,

Physical Culture School,

Festing Street,

HANLEY, N Staffs

Dr. ALLINSON FOR HEALTH.

MEDICAL ESSAYS, IN 5 VOLS.,

Vol. 1 contains Articles on Constipation, Biliousness, Eczema, Blackheads, Nervousness, Deafness, Itch, Worms, &c. Post free, 1s. 2d.

Vol. 2 contains Articles on the Hair, Want of Energy, Stoutness, Thinness, Children's Complaints, Anæmia, Bad Legs, Tumours, Diarrhœa, &c. Post free, 1s. 2d.

Vol. 3 contains Articles on Varicose Veins, Boils, Epilepsy, Mercurial Diseases, Wind, Stomach Troubles, &c. Post free, 1s. 2d.

Vol. 4 contains Articles on Sunstroke, Dog Bites, Lice, Quinsy, Shingles, Erysipelas, Ulcer of Stomach, Influenza, Psoriasis, &c. Post free, 1s. 2d.

Vol. 5 contains Articles on Training, Whitlow, Red Nose, Blushing and Flushing, Toothache, Inflamed Eyelids, Apoplexy, Wounds, Burns, Scalds, Bruises, &c. Post free, 1s. 2d.

A SYSTEM OF HYGIENIC MEDICINE ... 1s. 2d.
BOOK FOR MARRIED WOMEN ... 1s. 2d.
BOOK ON LUNG COMPLAINTS ... 1s. 2d.
PAMPHLETS TO YOUNG MEN ... 1s. 1d.
DIET and DIGESTION, post free ... 7d.
RHEUMATISM AND ITS CURE ... 7d.

All the above can be got from

Dr. T. R. ALLINSON, Ex. L.R.C.P. Ed.

433 Room, 4, Spanish Place,

MANCHESTER SQUARE, LONDON, W.

Consultation Hours—10 a.m. to 1 p.m. Fees 10s. 6d. 6 to 8 p.m. Fee 5s. Advice by Post. 5s.

STEMPEL'S GYMNASIUM and

Scientific Physical Training Institute. Est. 1883.

75, ALBANY ST., REGENT'S PARK, LONDON, N.W.

Finest Gymnasium in England.

Classes (ditto **Private**) for **Gentlemen, Ladies, Boys and Children. Fencing, Boxing, Wrestling.** Every branch of **Gymnastics, Calisthenics, Remedial Classes.**

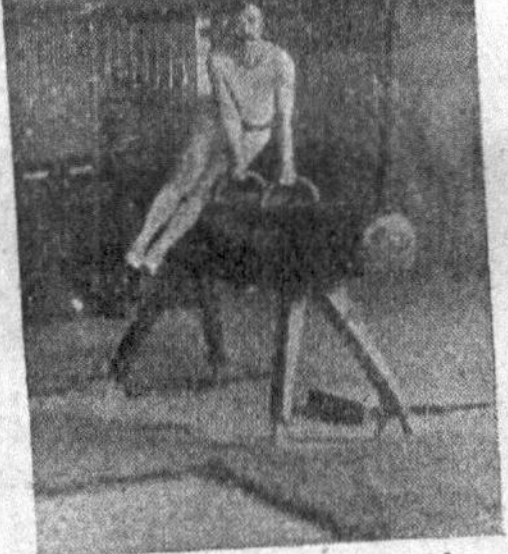

Medical Gymnastics,

Teachers Coached and Trained.

Ask for "General" also "Special Prospectus."

All Lessons and Classes under "Personal Direction of the Sole Propr. & Director **ADOLF A. STEMPEL, M.G.T.I.**

Largest Gymnastic Apparatus Depot in England. New Illustrated Catalogue of Gymnastic Apparatus free. All Apparatus on Stempel's Portable and Adjustable System. **Over 200** complete Gymnasia fitted up in this country.

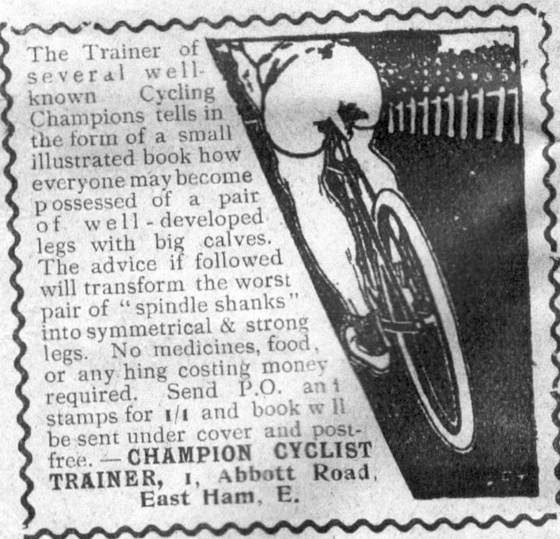

Sale and Exchange.

12 *Words for* 6d. (*minimum* 6d.)

First Volume.—Nos. 1 & 2 are out of print, but Nos. 3 to 12 inclusive, will be sent, post free, to any address in the United Kingdom for 1s. Abroad 1/6. All back Nos. of present volume can be supplied, post free, for 1½d. each. (August and September Nos. 2½d. each.)

Men of Muscle : All about them and their performances, by W. M. VARDON.—Sandow, Sampson, Topham, Weight-lifting extraordinary, Early Athletes, Feats of Gymnasts, &c., &c. Post free for six stamps. W. M. Vardon, 37, Myddelton Square, London, E.C.

Macfadden Exerciser, Style D, cost 8/6, sell for 4/6, including Instruction Book.—Wilton, c/o HEALTH AND STRENGTH Offices, 73, Farringdon Street E.C.

Sandow Developer, good order, 8s.—Smythe, c/o HEALTH AND STRENGTH Offices.

Wanted, Sandow's 12s. 6d book, also Sampson's book, and photos and prints of strong men.—Address particulars and prices to "Strongbow," c/o HEALTH AND STRENGTH Offices.

Wanted, heavy dumb-bells, bar-bells, ring weights, cheap, for cash :—"Instructor," c/o HEALTH AND STRENGTH Offices.

Instruction in Hand-balancing wanted by a novice. —MACKLIN, 50, Penton Place, Walworth.

"Strength," by Sandow, exchange for "Ideal Physical Culture," by Apollo.—JOHN O'HANLON, William Street, Portadown,

Wanted, Shot loading dumb-bell, about 50-lbs.— STEWART, 175, Northcote Road, Clapham, S.W.

Sandow Developer, Good working order, 7/6. G.P., care of HEALTH & STRENGTH.

Apollo's "Ideal Physical Culture" book, unsoiled, 1/11 postfree.—Workman, c/o HEALTH & STRENGTH. 73, Farringdon Street, E.C.

THE MACFADDEN EXERCISER

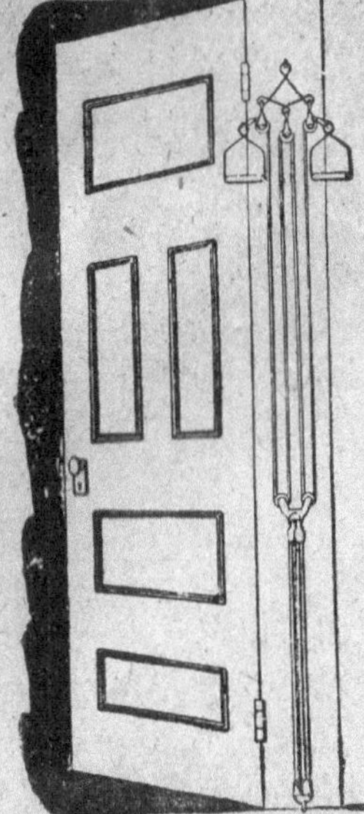

FIXED FOR USE ONE WAY
(or upside down).

can be put up without a tool—the screw hooks accompanying each outfit being sharp, gimlet pointed they can be screwed in any wood. The tension can be changed—made lighter or stronger—instantly. It is noiseless.

There is no conceivable motion that cannot be made on this exerciser. This gives you a complete gymnasium, right in your own home, at a small cost. It bears the stamp of an 1897 patent. The makers have had a chance to improve on all exercisers invented before theirs.

No other exerciser, with a rubber resistance, avoids entirely the direct, tenacious tension of rubber as this does. The outward pull is over twice as strong as the return pull, therefore the muscles are flexed while pulling outward, but relaxed when returning. The leading physical culture experts of the world have always objected to all rubber exercisers, because of their tenacious clinging tension, which is entirely avoided in this Exerciser. These experts claim that to secure the best physiological results from exercise, the flexed and relaxed condition of the muscles must follow in quick succession. Every time you flex a muscle you force the blood onward, and as it relaxes the blood flows in, and when rapidly flexed and reflexed a greatly accelerated circulation is created in every muscle thus used. You can readily understand that when the return pull of an exerciser, as on all entire rubber machines, is just as strong as the outward pull, the muscles will be flexed both ways, and that the muscles in action will be flexed during several movements while using exercisers of this character.

There is no expensive rubber cord running over pulleys — the Macfadden Exercisers are therefore more durable than the entire rubber machines. Instead of the wear being on a thin cord covering the rubber, as in the all-rubber exercisers, it is all on a solid braided cord.

PRICES:

Style A.
21/.
Postage 6d.

(With 128-page Instruction Book Fitted with cork handles and a very fine grade of heavy rubber. All metal parts heavily nickelled, fitted with four rubbers, adjustable to strength of anyone. Guaranteed one year.

Style B.
16/6
Postage 6d.

(With Instruction Book). Same pulleys as Style A. Metal parts nickelled, though not quite so finely finished; handles wood; strength of rubber 5-lbs. less than Style A. Guaranteed one year.

Style C
12/6
Postage 5d.

(With Instruction Book). Metal parts nickelled, with adjustable, silent-running, ebonised pulleys. three strands. Very strong and durable. Guaranteed six months.

Style D.
8/6
Postage 5d.

(With small Instruction Book) Wood pulleys; metal parts plain finish; strength from 3 to 25-lbs.

Extra Rubbers and Parts.

Single Rubber for C and D Outfits, 1s. each; for Style B, 1s. 3d. each; for Style A 1s. 6d. each; Postage 1d. extra. **Double Rubber** for Style C. and D Outfits, 2s. each; for Style B, 2s. 6d. each; for Style A, 3s. each. Postage 2d. extra. **Triple Rubber** for Style C and D Outfits 3s. each; for Style B, 4s. each; for Style A, 4s. 6d. each. Postage 2d. extra. **New Cords.** Style D, 3s.; C, 3s. 6d.; B. 4s.; A, 4s. 6d. Postage 2d. extra. Macfadden's Instruction Book 1s. Postage 2d.

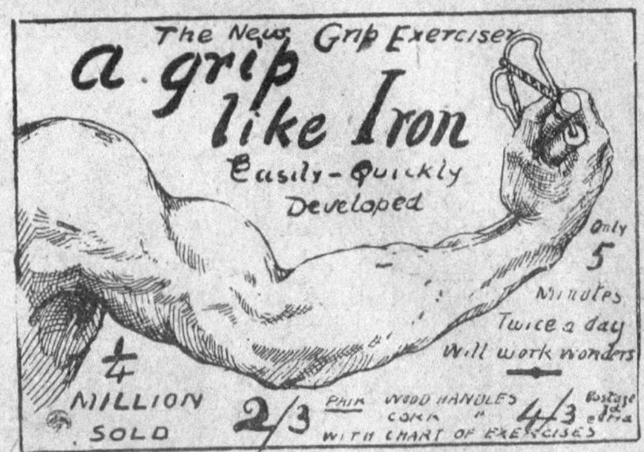

GRIP DEVELOPERS.

Ladies', Men's and Athletes' strengths supplied. Men's sent unless otherwise ordered. Athletes' strength 1s. per pair extra. Postage 3d.

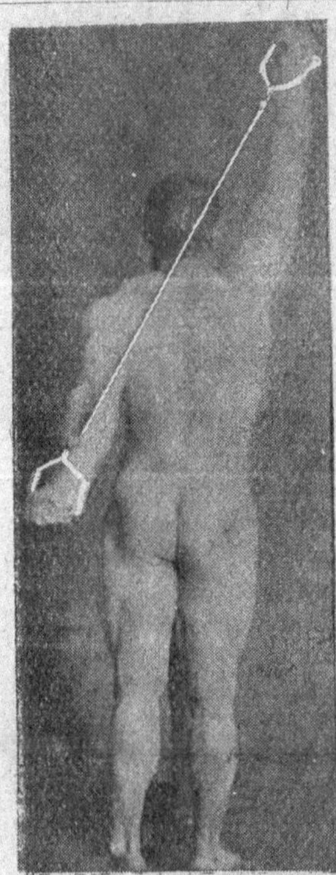

CHEST EXPANDER.

Broadens shoulders and Deepens Chest. Gives head and neck a fine poise. Develops Neck, Triceps & Chest Muscles.
Prices:

1 Rubber (children's) *2/6

2 Rubbers (juvenile's) *3/6

5 Rubbers (men's) †6/6

5 Rubbers (athletes') †7/6

5 Rubbers (extra strong athletes') †10/6

*Postage 3d.
†Postage 4d.

Call and inspect our goods. EVERYTHING FOR HEALTH AND STRENGTH. *No obligation to purchase.*

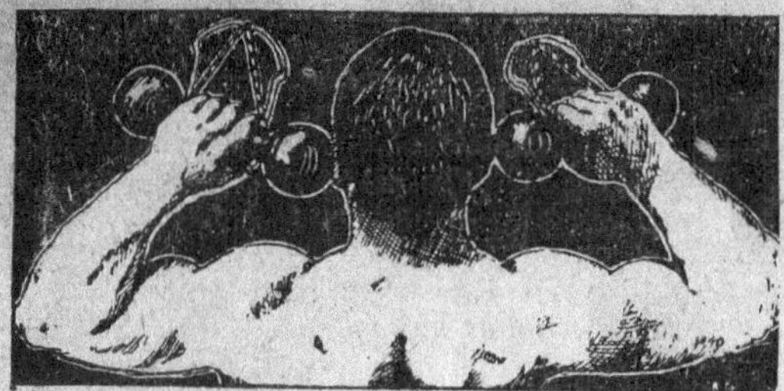

THE WIDE-GRIP DUMB-BELLS.

Combines the advantages of the Grip or Wrist Machine with that of the dumb-bell. Everyone who has developed strength by using the Wrist Machine will achieve further development by use of the Wide-Grip Dumb-bells. Weight about 2 lbs. each. Complete with chart of exercises.

Plain Wood ... ... 6s. 6d. pair. ⎰ Postage
Polished Rosewood... 8d. 6d. ,, ⎱ 6d.

Ladies', Men's and Athletes' strengths supplied. Men's sent unless otherwise ordered. Athletes' strength 1s. per pair extra.

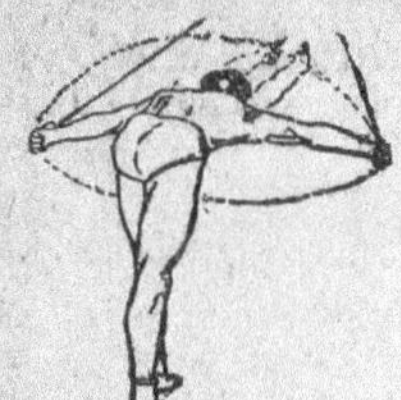

THE "HEALTH & STRENGTH" EXERCISER.

Works on one hook, is very light and handy, especially suitable for travellers. Complete with chart of exercises.

Price 3/6   Postage 3d.

Sandow's Developer.

Price 12/6, Post free.

Parts.—Pair of Sandow Pattern Dumb-bells, Detachable Screw Heads, perfect Balance, 4/6 per pair; Interchangeable Screw Heads for above (from 2-lbs. to 10-lbs.) 4d. per lb.; Extra Chest Expander Strands, 3/- per pair; Extra Long Strands for Weight Lifting, 4/- per pair; Chest Expander with Dumb-bells and Chart of Exercises, complete, 7/6; Chart of General Exercises, 1/6; Chart of Chest Expander Exercises 6d.

Whitely Health Exerciser.

Ladies' 4/6.   Men's 5/11.   Athletes' 6/11.
Postage 4d.

SANDOW'S GRIP DUMB-BELLS.

Greatly superior to old pattern Dumb-bells. Springs secure. A concentrated fixed grip during exercise. Complete with Chart of Exercises   Per pair

For Children, nickelled	...	...	...	5/-
,, Girls & Boys ,,	...	...	...	7/6
,, Ladies & Youths ...	...	...	...	10/6
,, Gentlemen ,, ...	...	...	...	12/6
,, ,, (enamelled) ...	...	...	...	7/6

Plain Dumb-bells,

1¾d. per lb.

Leather covered handles, 2-lbs. 1/3, 3-lbs. 1/9, 4-lbs. 2/=, 5-lbs. 2/6. 6-lbs. 2/9 per pair, Heavier at proportionate prices.
Nickel Plated, 6d. per lb.
Special Patterns, according to style and quantity.

DUMB-BELLS FOR STRONG MEN AND WEIGHT-LIFTERS.

HOLLOW, TO LOAD WITH SHOT.

Polished Wrought Steel Handles, with Swelled Grips and Wrought Collars at Ends, and fitted with Polished Nuts. Blacked Hollow Balls, each fitted with Screw-plug for Loading.

Diameter of Balls.	Weight Empty.	Weight Full.	Price Each.
5½ inches	17-lbs.	35-lbs	12/6
6 ,,	22 ,	45 ,,	15/=
7 ,,	37 ,,	80 ,,	20/=
8 ,,	56 ,,	130 ,,	25/=
9 ,,	68 ,,	180 ,,	30/=
10½ ,,	94 ,,	250 ,,	35/=
12 ,,	122 ,,	400 ,,	42/6
15 ,,	200 ,,	550 ,,	50/=

If with best finished Nickel-plated Handles and Nuts 4/6 each extra.

ESTIMATES FOR SPECIAL SIZES FREE.

Shot for Loading, in 28-lb. bags, 7/= per bag.

N.B.—The price of Shot fluctuates.

BAR-BELLS FOR STRONG MEN AND WEIGHT-LIFTERS.

HOLLOW, TO LOAD WITH SHOT.

Polished Wrought Steel Hollow Bars, one Swelled Grip in centre, Wrought Collars at ends, and fitted with Polished Nuts. Blacked Hollow Balls, each fitted with Screw-plug for Loading.

Diameter of Balls.	Weight Empty.	Weight Full.	Price Each. £ s. d.
7* inches	56-lbs.	110-lbs.	1 10 0
8 ,,	65 ,,	160 ,,	2 0 0
9 ,,	80 ,,	220 ,,	2 10 6
10½ ,,	105 ,,	300 ,,	3 0 0
12 ,,	156 ,,	415 ,,	4 5 0
15 ,,	215 ,,	600 ,,	5 0 0

*7 inch Bar-bells have no Grip, but are centre-marked. With 3 Swelled Grips on Bar, 5/= extra. With Nickel-plated Bar and Nuts, best finish—7 inch, 17/= extra; 8 and 9 inches 20/= extra; 10½, 12 and 15 inches, 24/= extra. ESTIMATES FOR SPECIAL SIZES FREE. Shot for Loading, in 28-lb. bags, 7/= per bag.
N.B.—The price of Shot fluctuates.

Iron Walking Sticks.

For Strengthening and Developing the Wrist and Forearm, and for Self Defence. Shepherd's Crook Pattern.

Weight— lbs.	2	3	4	5	6	7	8
Ebonized, plain	3/6	4/6	4/6	5/0	6/0	6/6	7/0
Japanned, imitation Hazel, Malacca, &c.	5/6	6/6	6/6	8/0	9/0	9/6	10/0
Covered, hand sewn nut brown leather, brass ferrule at end...	15/6	16/6	16/6	17/6	18/6	19/0	19/6

Weight—Lbs.	9	10	11	12	13	14	15
Ebonized, plain	7/6	8/0	8/0	8/6	8/6	9/0	9/6
Japanned. imitation Hazel, Malacca, &c.	10/6	11/0	11/0	11/6	12/0	12/6	13/0
Covered, hand sewn nut brown leather, brass ferrule at end...	20/0	20/6	20/6	21/0	21/0	21/6	22/0

Juggling Weights.

HOLLOW (CONICAL OR ROUND).

With Fixed Handle	16/6	each.
,, Loose Ring Handle	18/6	,,
,, ,, ,, Nickel-plated	23/6	,,

,, Weight, Empty, 56-lbs.; loading up to 100-lbs.

Catching Weights (HOLLOW).

With Fixed Polished Crown Handle ...	16/6	each.
Nickel-plated Handle extra	4/6	,,

Weight, Empty, 32-lbs.; loading up to 100-lbs.

Conical weights in sections, square weights, ring-shot, triangular, oval or special shape handles, loose or fixed, polished or nickelled, and special sizes and weights. Prizes on application.

SHOT MEASURE AND INJECTOR.

For filling hollow dumb-bells and bar-bells with any desired weight. Price **3/=**. Postage 3d.

PUTTING SHOTS.

Blacked, 16-lbs. weight ... ... each **4/=**

THROWING HAMMERS.

Solid Ball Heads and Ash Handles, 17-lbs. weight ... ... each **8/6**

FINGER SPRINGS.

Steel, for strengthening Fingers & Hands, each **2/6**
Leather-covered Centres, extra.

ARM RINGS.

For Hardening the Biceps and Triceps Muscles, in polished steel, any size ... each **5/=**

Cannon Balls, Roman Columns, Lifting Machines.

Wickerwork "Surprise" Bar-bells,

To put One Man Inside each Ball. 30 inches diameter; 8 feet long; weight 56-lbs. Steel Chains, Bars, Links, &c., and Every description of Iron-work, &c., for Professional Strong Men, estimated for and made to order.

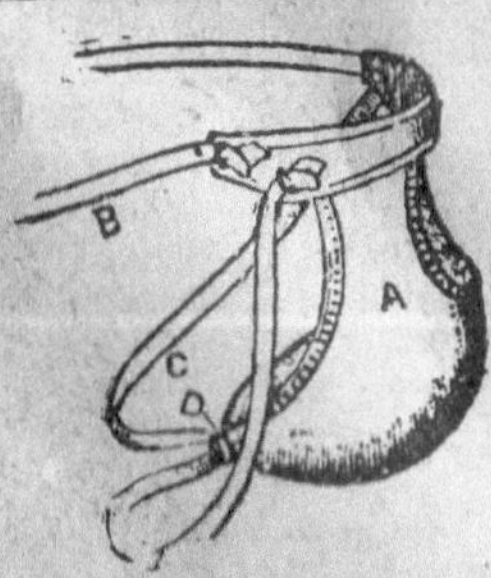

THE HEALTH AND STRENGTH SUSPENSORY

Is used by thousands, including a large number of doctors, those engaged in arduous work, whilst those who are constrained to walk, stand or sit for some time will find our Suspensory a wonderful Support. Athletes especially appreciate our Suspensories because they prevent rupture, twist and chafing.

PRICES AND DESCRIPTIONS.

one	two	POUCH.	WAIST BAND	LEG BAND
1/6	2/9	Cotton.	Non-Elastic	Part Elastic
2/=	3/9	,,	,,	Elastic
3/=	5/6	,,	Elastic	,,
4/=	7/3	Silk.	,,	,,
5/=	8/9	Silk ,, net	,,	,,

SIZES.—We keep in stock three sizes; Large, Medium, and Small. Medium size sent unless other size or height mentioned.

Every Suspensory is sent carefully packed free from observation.

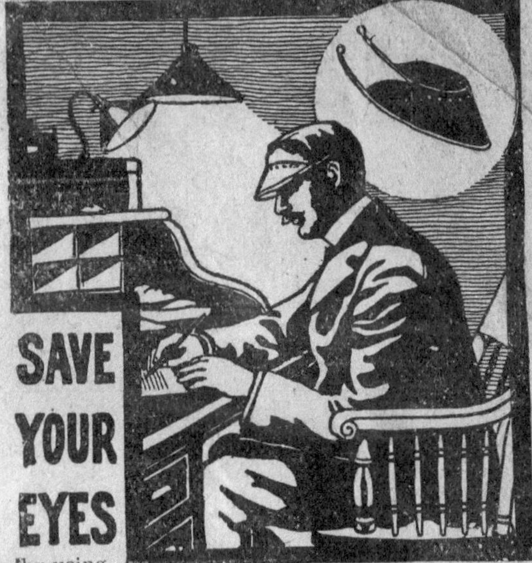

by using the HEALTH & STRENGTH **EYE SHADE** when reading or working with artificial light. Made of patent semi-transparent material, it holds itself in position. Price 1/6, with valuable "Eyesight Advice," in box, 1/6 post free.

FRICTION TOWEL. Promotes the healthy circulation of the blood. A fine tonic aid to, and doubling the value of, a bath. Price **3/6** each. Postage 4d.

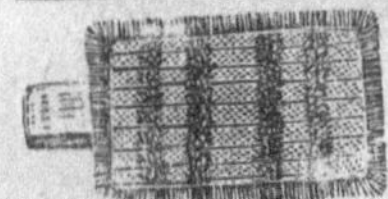

HORSEHAIR PAD. A cheap form of horsehair brush. Last for years. Wet or dry use. Price **1/6.** Postage 2d.

HORSEHAIR FLESH GLOVES, woven in a most peculiar manner on to a foundation of special cloth. Made in two "strengths," *medium* and *soft*. The experience of a brisk "rub down" with a pair of these horsehair flesh gloves should not be missed. Circulation is roused and a fine feeling of exhilaration remains for the rest of the day—affording a natural development of vital force.

Price **5/=** per pair. Postage 3d.

HORSEHAIR BATH GLOVES. (For wet or dry use).

Very durable, healthful and refreshing. A luxurious addition to a Turkish or warm bath. **3/6** each. Postage 3d.

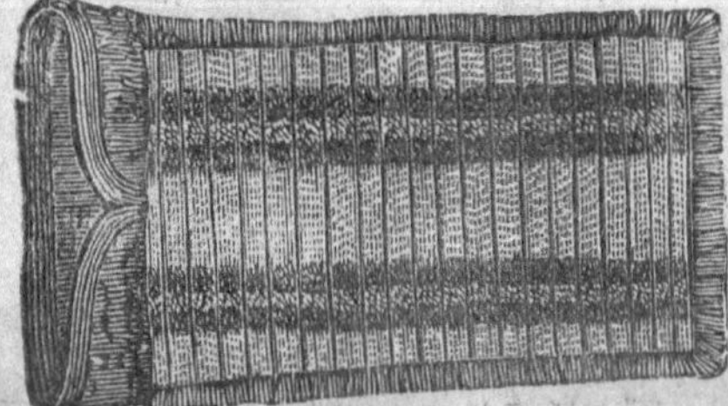

HAND BRUSH, for polishing skin and stimulating capillary circulation. Has hand strap. Real Siberian pigs' bristles. Will last for years. Satinwood-finish back. Price **5/=.** Postage 3d.

The HEALTH & STRENGTH HYGIENIC TOOTH BRUSH,

1/-

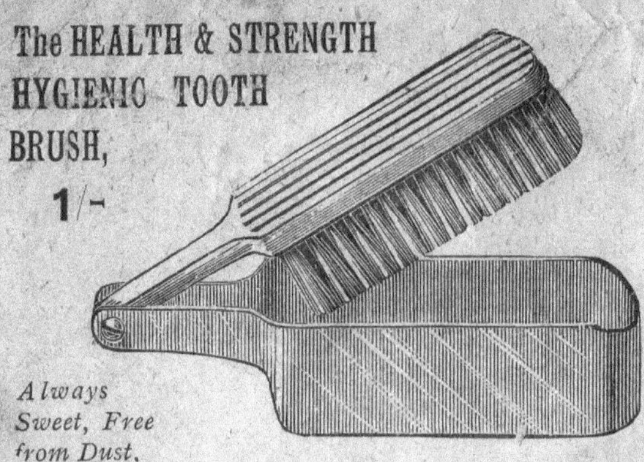

Always Sweet, Free from Dust.

Unlike the ordinary tooth brush the bristles are not set close together, consequently it is impossible for decaying particles of food, tartar and other deposits to collect. The arrangement of the bristles in the Health & Strength Tooth Brush also ensures the thorough cleaning of the teeth. The *separate* sets of bristles *enter* and clean crevices. A solid face of bristles simply slides *over*. When not in use brush portion can be folded into nickelled case, protecting bristles from dust, etc. Case has small holes for draining brush. When folded our Tooth Brush takes up smaller space than any other on the market, making it eminently suitable for travellers

Price, 1/= each.   Postage 1d.

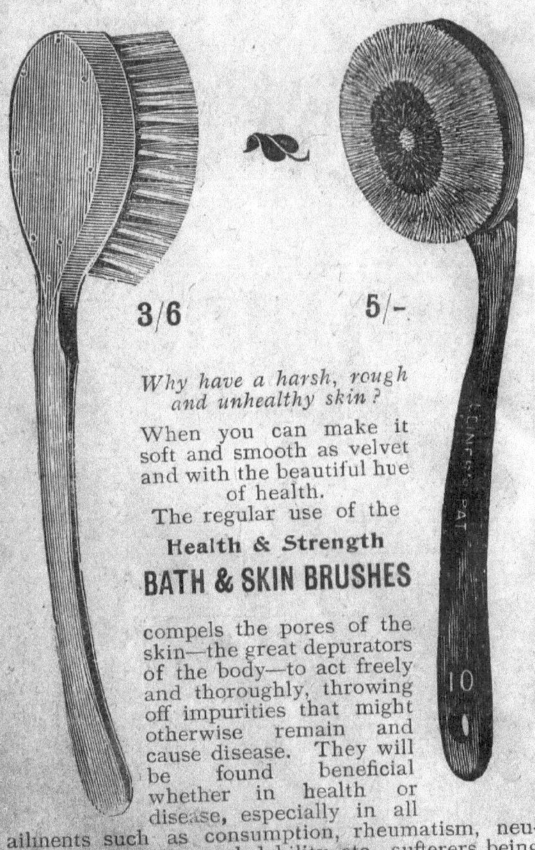

3/6   **5/-**

Why have a harsh, rough and unhealthy skin?

When you can make it soft and smooth as velvet and with the beautiful hue of health.

The regular use of the

Health & Strength
BATH & SKIN BRUSHES

compels the pores of the skin—the great depurators of the body—to act freely and thoroughly, throwing off impurities that might otherwise remain and cause disease. They will be found beneficial whether in health or disease, especially in all ailments such as consumption, rheumatism, neuralgia, catarrh, general debility, etc., sufferers being materially assisted towards recovery by their use.

HAIR CULTURE BRUSHES & COMB.

(IN LEATHER CASE AS ILLUSTRATED).

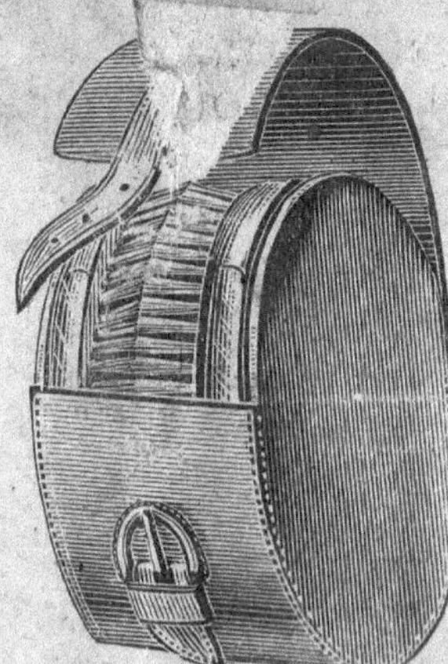

Unlike most hair brushes, the knots of bristles in these brushes are not set close together. The brush, therefore, does not collect scurf, dust, etc., whilst the bristles also are more penetrative in use. White Comb with well cut teeth. Case, best glossy brown cowhide.   Price **5/=.** Postage 3d.

GOOD HEALTH, or, The Physiology of Dietetics and Massage.

By F. C. IRELAND, B.Sc. Food is the fuel of the human system, and has the most important bearing on health. Price 2/6 net. Postage 4d.

"MACFADDEN'S NEW HAIR CULTURE."—"*No excuse for becoming bald.*" Strong luxuriant hair, how to develop it. No oils—no drugs—simply a natural remedy based on physiological laws as accurately fixed as the laws governing development of muscular system. Post free (under cover) for **4/=.**

LUNG GYMNASTICS

And the Art of Breathing, The proper aeration of the life blood is one of the secrets of a long and healthy life. Price **2/10.** post free.

LIGHT DUMB-BELLS.

By the Director of the famous Woolwich Polytechnic Gymnasium. Photographic Pictures of Exercises. This work has had the largest sale of any book on dumb-bells. Sent by return post for only **7**d. stamps; or with **1/-** book on Indian Clubs, **1/6**, post free.

STRAIGHT TALK from one of the cleverest **WHO** specialist doctors America has ever produced. The "Talk" occupies nearly 1,000 pages, and is vitally interesting, important and **SHOULD** useful to every man who is married, or expects to be. 200 life-coloured plates. Largest circulation of any book ever published next to the Bible. Over 1,000,000 **NOT** copies sold, and selling in ever-increasing quantities daily. Ours is the genuine, unabridged, American edition, with coloured plates, **MARRY?** etc. Sealed free from observation, and post free 6/6.

THE ATHLETE'S CONQUEST, or, The Romance of an Athlete. A stirring Novel by Prof. B. A. MACFADDEN, the famous American Strong Man, Lecturer and Author. Author of "Macfadden's Physical Training. Price **1/2**, post free.

WHAT A YOUNG HUSBAND OUGHT

concerning himself, his wife, and his children. Strength, weakness, social vice, the organs, personal purity, the prevalence of disease—the beginning, progress, and end—how to avoid; selection of a wife.   Post free, 4/6. **TO KNOW**